High Blood Pressure Lowered Naturally

Your Arteries Can Clean Themselves!

Publisher's Note

This book is for information only. It does not constitute medical advice and should not be construed as such. We cannot guarantee the safety or effectiveness of any drug, treatment, or advice mentioned. Some of these tips may not be effective for everyone.

A good doctor is the best judge of what medical treatment may be needed for certain conditions and diseases. We recommend in all cases that you contact your personal doctor or health care provider before taking or discontinuing any medications, or before treating yourself in any way

I have told you these things, so that in me you will have peace. In this world you will have trouble. But take heart! I have overcome the world.

John 16:33 (NIV)

FC&A Medical Publishing®
103 Clover Green
Peachtree City, GA 30269

Produced by the staff of FC&A

ISBN 978-1-932470-24-6

Table of Contents

Introduction

What do you think is the number one health problem today? When asked that question, most people answer "cancer." Most people are wrong. The number one cause of death in men and women is heart disease and has been since 1900.

Why has heart disease become such a common killer? Partly because modern inventions — cars, remote controls, elevators — have made people more sedentary. You may have rolled your eyes when your grandfather told you he walked five miles barefoot in the snow to get to school, but the fact is, he probably walked a lot more than you do. He probably had to. Although everyone knows exercise builds strong muscles, and your heart is a muscle, more than 60 percent of the people don't exercise at the recommended levels.

Life expectancy rates have increased dramatically in this century, due mostly to the miracles of modern medicine like antibiotics, vaccinations, and better prenatal care. However, this increased life expectancy may actually contribute to heart disease's title as number one killer. People aren't dying young from other causes, which means they live long enough to damage their hearts.

Scientists have learned a lot in the last century about nutrition and how it affects your health. Nevertheless, many people today rely on highly processed, fat-laden foods. These high-fat diets contribute to high cholesterol, which is a risk factor for heart disease. Excess weight is also hard on your heart. Maintaining an ideal body weight may reduce your risk of heart disease by 35 to 55 percent.

The biggest contributing factor to high rates of heart disease is smoking. This is one luxury of modern living you can definitely live without. Smoking accounts for about 21 percent of all heart disease deaths. If you're a smoker, quitting now can reduce your risk of heart disease 50 to 70 percent in the next five years. It will also reduce your risk of the second leading killer disease — cancer.

Researchers and doctors are working hard to control heart disease, and they are making great progress. Although the death toll from the disease has declined 54 percent over the last three decades, it's still the number one health problem.

To prevent heart disease from adding you to the statistics, take charge of your own health. Dr. William Castelli, director of the Framingham Heart Study, says that fully 75 percent of heart disease can be prevented by dietary and lifestyle changes.

The *High Blood Pressure Lowered Naturally* provides information to help you make those changes. In the following pages, you'll find advice about nutrition, exercise, stress management, and other heart-healthy lifestyle strategies. By using this information to keep your heart healthy, you just may add years to your life.

Leading causes of death

	Males	Females
Heart disease	36.2%	43.3%
Cancer	22.9%	21.9%
Accidents	5.4%	2.9%

How Your Heart Works

Blueprint for a healthy heart

Close your fist and look at it. That's about the size of your heart. It's not very large, but that little muscular organ does a king-sized job in pumping blood all over your body.

Now put your hand over your heart, like you're reciting a pledge. You're probably off the mark just a little. It's located only slightly left of the center of your chest, between your lungs, and probably a little lower than you might think.

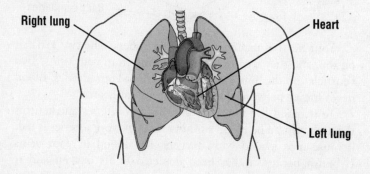

Right lung   Heart

Left lung

3

Your heart's closeness to your lungs is no accidental arrangement. The two organs work together to supply your body with the oxygen it needs to survive. The right side of your heart sends blood to your lungs, where it receives oxygen and gets rid of carbon dioxide, which is a waste product. The left side of your heart takes in the newly oxygenated blood from your lungs and pumps it to the rest of your body. As the blood travels through your body, it delivers oxygen and picks up carbon dioxide.

Your circulating blood follows a path that resembles a figure eight. The right side of the loop represents circulation to your lungs and back to your heart, and the left side of the loop represents circulation to your body.

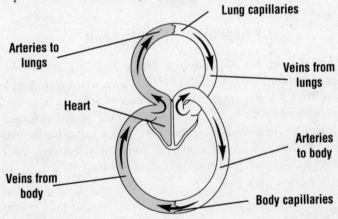

Your heart is made up of four chambers. The two atria sit on top, and they receive blood returning from your veins. Two ventricles on the bottom pump blood into your arteries. Blood never moves between the two sides of your heart.

Your blood leaves your heart through arteries and returns through veins. The blood running through your arteries is red, because it is loaded with oxygen. The blood in your veins is bluish because it has been depleted of its oxygen and is carrying waste products instead. The pulmonary veins are exceptions. They carry newly oxygenated blood from the lungs to the left atrium.

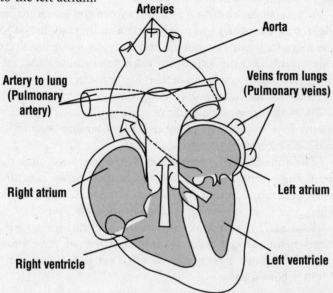

The blood your heart sends coursing through your body every minute of the day does more than deliver oxygen and pick up carbon dioxide. It also carries hormones from your glands to wherever they are needed. Waste products other than carbon dioxide are delivered to your kidneys and liver, where they are neutralized. Blood also picks up nutrients from your intestines and takes them to the rest of your body. No wonder your heart is critical for survival.

And the beat goes on ...

You can't see your heart, but you know it's working by its beat. A healthy adult heart beats between 60 and 100 times per minute when you're resting. To find out your resting heart rate, place two fingers on the inside of your wrist, until you can feel your pulse. Using a watch with a second hand, count the beats for 10 seconds and multiply by six.

You know your heart rate increases when you get excited or frightened, like when you're watching a really scary movie. It also increases when you exercise and decreases when you sleep. Other things that can affect your heart rate include stress, caffeine, tobacco, alcohol, and certain medications.

Your average heart rate tends to slow down as you age. It may also slow down as a result of athletic training. Your heart doesn't have to pump as many times in a minute because it's pumping more strongly with each beat.

The time from the beginning of one heartbeat until the beginning of the next is called the cardiac cycle. The time when the heart is contracting is called the systole, and the time when your heart is relaxing is called the diastole.

Your heart has to relax fully in order to fill back up with blood before it contracts again. Each beat of your heart pumps out about 3 ounces of blood. That adds up to about 2,000 gallons a day.

Heart Disorders

Safeguard your heart from these 4 enemies

Almost half of the men who die suddenly of heart disease don't have any previous evidence of disease. If you're aware that you have a heart problem, consider yourself lucky. You have time to get help and make some lifestyle changes.

Heart disease can affect any part of your cardiovascular system — which includes your heart and blood vessels. It's possible to have more than one type of heart disease at once, and sometimes one condition leads to another. For example, you may develop atherosclerosis, which could lead to angina, or a nonfatal heart attack could cause congestive heart failure.

To safeguard your heart from disease, learn all you can about your heart and blood vessels and their common problems.

Atherosclerosis. Your arteries have to be strong and elastic to withstand the pressure of your heart pumping blood throughout your body. As you get older, your arteries gradually become less flexible, just like the rest of your body.

Atherosclerosis affects mostly your major arteries, including your coronary arteries. The walls of these arteries become thicker and irregular, and plaques form, slowing down the flow of blood.

7

Although atherosclerosis can happen to anyone, certain things make you more susceptible. A high-fat diet, smoking, high blood pressure, high cholesterol levels, a sedentary lifestyle, and diabetes can make you more likely to develop atherosclerosis.

Arrhythmia. Most of the time, your heart beats steady as a clock, but every once in a while, you feel a quick fluttering, or your heart "skips a beat." This is called arrhythmia, and usually, it's nothing to worry about. It happens to everyone now and then.

Some arrhythmias are caused by stress, tobacco, caffeine, alcohol, or certain medications, while others are a symptom of heart disease. Sometimes, the arrhythmias themselves can be dangerous.

When your heart beats too slowly, it is called bradycardia. With this condition, your heart may slow down too much and just stop beating. It may be a symptom of an underlying disease, or it could mean your heart medication, such as a beta blocker, is slowing your heartbeat too much.

When your heartbeat is too fast, it is called tachycardia. This can be caused by stress, too much caffeine, or certain types of medication, especially diet pills. While everyone's heartbeat speeds up occasionally, if you have episodes of tachycardia often, or if the episodes last longer than a few minutes, see your doctor. He can help get your heartbeat back on track.

Don't panic if your heart flutters or races once in a while. For most people, this is completely harmless, but if you're concerned, see your doctor.

Angina pectoris. Chest pain, or angina, is the most common symptom of heart disease. The pain of angina is a sign your heart isn't getting enough blood, which means it isn't getting enough oxygen.

Although angina is painful, it's nature's way of warning you to take care of your heart. Making some lifestyle changes, like getting regular exercise; eating low-fat, high-fiber foods; managing stress; and stopping smoking would be a good place to start. If you stop the angina, you may be able to head off a heart attack. But remember — check with your doctor before starting an exercise plan.

Angina is usually triggered by too much stress, too much to eat, or too much exercise, but it can occur when you're resting. A healthy heart can handle the extra demands created by "overdoing," but an unhealthy one can't.

Don't assume chest pain always means you have heart disease. There are many causes of chest pain, including indigestion and heartburn. But if your chest hurts for more than a few minutes, or if the pain is sudden and severe, don't hesitate to call for emergency help. You could be having a heart attack.

Congestive heart failure. This doesn't mean your heart has just decided to quit working. Heart failure occurs when your heart fails to pump enough blood to meet your body's demands. This disease is fairly common, affecting one out of every 100 people in the United States.

The first symptoms of heart failure are usually fatigue and weakness. If your condition continues, you may experience breathing difficulties and your legs, feet, and ankles may swell. This swelling is where the "congestive" part of heart failure comes in. It's caused by blood backing up into your veins, forcing fluid out of your blood vessels and into surrounding tissue. This backup of fluid can also cause your liver and other internal organs to become enlarged.

Fortunately, congestive heart failure can be treated with diuretics or other medications. You'll also find many natural suggestions for dealing with heart failure throughout this book.

🐜 🐜 🐜

A 'bug' may cause heart disease

The causes of heart disease are many and varied — heredity, obesity, not enough exercise, homocysteine, cholesterol, smoking, and so on. Now researchers have uncovered a new possibility — one that may explain why many heart disease victims have no known risk factors.

Your heart disease may be caused by a "bug," a bacterium called *Chlamydia pneumoniae,* which is an infectious organism that can cause pneumonia, bronchitis, and sinus infections.

Researchers discovered that plaques from the arteries of people with coronary heart disease contained unusually high levels of this bacteria. One study found that antibiotics significantly reduced complications in people with severe heart disease.

While all this suggests that a bacterial infection may be the cause of heart disease in some people, more studies are needed to confirm this theory. However, researchers are excited by the prospect of someday being able to treat heart disease with antibiotics.

ℰ ℰ

How to survive a heart attack

You're sitting in your favorite easy chair watching a movie and snacking on popcorn when you get a severe pain in your chest. You wonder if you're having a heart attack or just an attack of indigestion.

A heart attack occurs when the blood flow to your heart stops or is greatly reduced. This happens because one of the arteries leading to your heart becomes blocked by a buildup of plaque or a blood clot. The medical term for a heart attack is myocardial infarction. An infarct is an area of tissue that has been permanently damaged from lack of oxygen.

The longer your heart is deprived of oxygen, the more likely you are to die or have permanent damage to your heart. The sooner you get medical help after a heart attack begins, the better your chances are for a full recovery.

Unfortunately, sudden death is sometimes the first symptom of a heart attack. Recognizing other symptoms may be the key to surviving. If you have any combination of the following symptoms, get emergency help immediately.

- Intense chest pain that lasts longer than a few minutes. The pain is often described as a squeezing feeling or a feeling of heavy pressure.

- Pain that spreads from your chest to your left arm and shoulder, back, or even your jaw.

- Shortness of breath.

- Lightheadedness or fainting.

- Nausea or vomiting.

- Heavy sweating.

If you think you are having a heart attack, call for help and then take an aspirin. A huge international study found that aspirin given to heart attack victims when admitted to the hospital decreased deaths significantly. It also reduced subsequent nonfatal heart attacks and strokes by almost half. The sooner aspirin was given, the greater the chances for recovery.

Here's the scoop on heart medications

Angina. Nitrates are commonly prescribed for angina. They work by relaxing or dilating all the blood vessels in your body. This helps move blood out of your heart and into your blood vessels, reducing your heart's demand for oxygen and easing angina pain. Nitroglycerin is probably the most familiar of the nitrates, and it comes in three forms — tablet, spray, and patch. You don't swallow the tablet, you place it under your tongue until it dissolves. The spray is also used under your tongue. For prolonged release, your doctor will probably recommend the patch.

Beta blockers are also prescribed for angina. They work by slowing your heartbeat and reducing your blood pressure. Because your heart beats fewer times per minute, its need for oxygen is lessened. Side effects of beta blockers include fatigue, dizziness, insomnia, and impotence.

Calcium channel blockers may also be prescribed for angina. They reduce heart rate, lower blood pressure, dilate your arteries, and decrease the strength of your heart's contractions. Other drug alternatives may be a better first-choice treatment for high blood pressure until the results of the latest studies are available. See the *High blood pressure* chapter for more information and cautions on calcium channel blockers.

Arrhythmia. Antiarrhythmics work by slowing nerve impulses in your heart and acting directly on heart tissue. Different types have different side effects, but the most common ones are stomach upset, trembling, dry mouth, blurry vision, and dizziness.

Congestive heart failure. The medicines most commonly prescribed for heart failure are Angiotensin Converting Enzyme (ACE) inhibitors and diuretics. See the *High blood pressure* chapter for more information about these medicines.

Blood vessel problems. Your doctor might prescribe anticoagulants if you are at high risk for having a heart attack or stroke. These medicines work by reducing the ability of your blood to form clots. The most common kind is warfarin (Coumadin). Antiplatelet medicines, like dipyridamole, and aspirin also help prevent blood clots.

Commonly prescribed heart medications

Angina	nitroglycerin (Nitrostat, Nitrogard)
	isosorbide dinitrate (Isordil, Sorbitrate, Dilatrate-SR)
	erythrityl tetranitrate (Cardilate)
	beta blockers and calcium channel blockers (See the ***High blood pressure*** chapter)
Heart failure	bumetanide (Bumex)
	ethacrynic (Edecrin)
	furosemide (Lasix)
	digoxin (Lanoxin, Lanoxicaps)
	ACE inhibitors (See the ***High blood pressure*** chapter)
Arrhythmia	quinidine (Cardioquin, Quinidex)
	procainamide (Procan SR)
	flecainide (Tambocor)
	disopyramide (Norpace)
	mexiletine (Mexitil)
	phenytoin (Dilantin)
Other	warfarin (Coumadin)
	aspirin
	dipyridamole (Persantine)

Protect yourself from dangerous drug interactions

Heart medications can help you, but if you're not aware of possible food or drug interactions, your medication may just make things worse.

If you're taking an anticoagulant like warfarin (Coumadin), stay away from NSAIDs, like aspirin and ibuprofen, and acetaminophen (Tylenol). These medicines also prevent blood clots, but taken together, they may thin your blood too much or cause internal bleeding. The same thing can happen if you take large doses of vitamin E. Eating large amounts of foods high in vitamin K, like spinach, broccoli, turnip greens, brussels sprouts, cauliflower, chick peas, and beef liver, can have the opposite effect. Too much vitamin K can decrease the effectiveness of anticoagulants. You don't have to stop eating these foods. Just maintain a balanced diet and avoid eating large amounts of them.

If your doctor prescribes beta-blockers or ACE inhibitors for your blood pressure, tell him if you regularly take NSAIDs for arthritis or other pain. NSAIDs can interfere with your blood pressure medication, which means you may need to have it monitored more closely.

If you're taking quinidine or digoxin, don't start taking the drug cimetidine (Tagamet) for ulcers. It increases the amount of these medicines absorbed by your body. This can result in dangerous arrhythmias.

High-fiber foods are good for your cholesterol levels, but they can slow down your body's ability to absorb certain medicines, including digoxin. And grapefruit juice can have the opposite effect, increasing the absorption of some medicines, particularly calcium channel blockers.

ﾞ🐜 ﾞ🐜 ﾞ🐜

Extreme weather hazardous to your heart

Weather that is too hot or too cold can affect your heart. When it's hot, your body sweats to cool off and you lose fluid, which decreases your blood volume. Your heart has to work harder to pump the reduced amount of blood through your body. Then, if you exercise outdoors in hot weather, you're doubling the strain on your heart.

You should know the symptoms of heat exhaustion and heatstroke and take steps immediately to cool yourself down. Heatstroke can be fatal.

Symptoms of heat exhaustion include heavy sweating; cold, clammy skin; dizziness; rapid heartbeat; headache; and nausea. If heat exhaustion progresses to heatstroke, your body, including your heart and brain, will begin to shut down completely. A high fever, slow pulse, low blood pressure, gray skin, and confusion are some of the symptoms of heatstroke.

Weather that is too cold can result in hypothermia, or a severely reduced body temperature. This happens because your body can't produce enough energy to keep your internal temperature warm enough. Symptoms of this potentially fatal condition include confusion, sleepiness, and lack of coordination. Heart failure is the most common cause of death in cases of hypothermia.

Protect yourself from hypothermia in cold weather by wearing layers of clothing and a hat and gloves. Also, don't drink alcohol before going out into the cold. You may think it's warming you up, but it's actually drawing warmth from your internal organs to your skin, making you more vulnerable to hypothermia.

❧ ❧

If surgery is your only option

No matter what kind of surgery you're having, there are some things you need to know to make your surgery a success:

❧ Ask if there are different ways of doing the surgery you're scheduled for. Some methods involve more extensive operations than others. Ask your doctor why he chose his method.

❧ Find out where you'll have your surgery. Most surgeons use one or two local hospitals. Ask your doctor if he knows how many operations like the one you're scheduled for have been performed in that hospital. If he doesn't know, call the hospital administration office and ask. Also ask about the hospital's success rates with this particular operation. The reason for making this extra effort is that some hospitals have higher success rates in certain operations than others. You want to use the hospital with the best success rate. However, some surgeries are now done on an outpatient basis, either in the doctor's office or in a special day surgery unit. If your doctor says you'll be having surgery as an outpatient, ask if that surgery is normally done on an outpatient basis. If not, ask why you'll be undergoing that surgery as an outpatient. You want to be in the right place for your operation.

- Have your doctor completely and clearly explain the surgery. Ask him what will happen to you before, during, and after your operation. Find out what kind of supplies, equipment, or any other help you'll need after surgery. Knowing exactly what to expect will help calm your fears and worries. Generally, the fewer anxieties and worries you have, the faster your body will heal.

- Ask your doctor about taking aspirin and any medicines that contain aspirin. Most of the time, your doctor will want you to stop taking these drugs at least a week before surgery. You should also ask your doctor what he wants you to do about other medicines you take regularly. Finally, let your doctor know if you drink or smoke regularly because these habits can affect the anesthesia.

- Don't eat or drink anything after midnight the night before your surgery. This is the general rule for people having surgery, but check with your doctor just in case. Some people are allowed to have clear liquids up to a few hours before they receive anesthesia.

- Arrange for a responsible adult to take you home after your surgery. Unless your surgery involves only local anesthesia, you won't be allowed to drive yourself home.

◆ Dress for comfort. Wear loose-fitting clothes and leave your valuables at home.

10 best hospitals for heart surgery

Just like doctors, some hospitals rate better than others. It's in your best interest to get treatment at the best hospital you can find. The more serious the problem, the better the hospital you'll want to be in. According to *U.S. News and World Report*, these hospitals are leading the way with the latest innovations in heart surgery.

Cleveland Clinic

Mayo Clinic, Rochester, Minn.

Brigham and Women's Hospital, Boston

Duke University Medical Center, Durham, N.C.

Massachusetts General Hospital, Boston

Johns Hopkins Hospital, Baltimore

Emory University Hospital, Atlanta

Texas Heart Institute at St. Luke's Episcopal Hospital, Houston

Stanford Hospital and Clinics, Stanford, Calif.

Barnes-Jewish Hospital, St. Louis

§▲ §▲ §▲

Cure worse than the disease

A recently published study supported the fact that heart surgery may be one cure that is worse than the disease. Almost 1,000 people who had suffered the most common type of heart attack were randomly chosen to undergo either invasive treatment or noninvasive treatment.

The people in the invasive group were tested by angiography, a procedure in which dye is injected through a tube into the coronary arteries, revealing the amount of blockage on an X-ray. They were then treated by balloon angioplasty or bypass surgery.

The people in the other group were tested by less-dangerous methods and treated with medication — no surgery. And guess what? The people who underwent invasive treatment, including surgery, were significantly more likely to die or have another heart attack than those who didn't have surgery. The surgery group was more than twice as likely to die or have another heart attack.

If your doctor thinks surgery is your only option, ask about a new, less-invasive surgery called keyhole bypass surgery.

Unlike standard bypass surgery, surgeons operate through a small incision instead of cutting through the breastbone. Because the surgeon doesn't have to stop the heart, a heart-lung bypass machine isn't necessary. The heart continues to beat on its own.

This less-invasive bypass surgery may reduce complications and death rates in high-risk patients.

Cholesterol

4 basic strategies to lower your cholesterol

You think you're as healthy as a horse — until the doctor's office calls with the results of your physical, and you find out your cholesterol is pushing 300.

A high cholesterol level is a warning that your heart is headed for trouble, but you can do something about it.

Snack to your heart's content. Don't be afraid to snack several times a day on low-fat foods, such as yogurt, fruit, vegetables, bagels, and whole-grain breads and cereals. As a matter of fact, evidence points to lower cholesterol levels in people who eat small meals several times a day. Eating often keeps hormones like insulin from rising and signaling your body to make cholesterol. Just make sure your total intake of calories doesn't go up when you eat more often.

Eat less saturated fat. You get cholesterol from two sources. Your body manufactures most of it in your liver, but you get dietary cholesterol from animal products, such as meat, dairy foods, and eggs. Plant foods, like vegetables, grains, and nuts, don't have any cholesterol.

While eating less cholesterol may help, the biggest dietary change you can make is to reduce your intake of saturated fat. Too much saturated fat can raise your cholesterol levels. Animal fats, like butter and lard, and some vegetable fats, like palm oil and coconut oil, are saturated. Substituting a liquid vegetable oil, like canola, when you're cooking is a good way to lower saturated fat in your diet. Here's a general guideline — the more saturated a fat is, the more solid it is at room temperature. You don't have to cut fat out of your diet altogether. Researchers say moderate decreases in fat intake can substantially lower cholesterol.

Get some exercise. Exercise can help you increase your good HDL cholesterol level and lower your bad LDL cholesterol. It also helps you lose weight and control diabetes and high blood pressure. And when you exercise, you are conditioning your heart along with your other muscles. All that adds up to good news for your heart.

Maintain a healthy weight. If you are overweight, lose weight. Weight loss lowers triglycerides, LDL, and VLDL cholesterol and raises HDL cholesterol. Researchers found that losing weight can increase your HDL cholesterol regardless of how much you exercise. If you exercise and lose weight, you will increase your HDL even more.

Understanding this powerful predictor of heart disease

Cholesterol is a soft, waxy substance that travels through your bloodstream. It helps form cell membranes and other tissues, as well as some hormones. Your body needs cholesterol, but too much can clog your arteries and lead to heart disease and stroke.

About half of the people in the United States have cholesterol levels at least slightly above the desirable level of 200. According to a recent study, lowering that figure by just 10 percent would result in a 20 percent decrease in heart attack deaths.

Cholesterol is a type of fat or lipid, and it can't dissolve in your blood like some nutrients. It has to be transported by carrier molecules, called lipoproteins. There are several types of lipoproteins, but the ones you hear the most about are low density lipoprotein (LDL) and high density lipoprotein (HDL).

Low density lipoprotein is the main cholesterol carrier in your blood. It's known as the "bad" cholesterol. If you have too much LDL cholesterol, it can build up on the walls of your arteries and combine with other substances to form a hard deposit called plaque. Plaque can make your arteries so narrow your heart has trouble pumping blood through them. A blood clot can also form near the site of the plaque. If it blocks the flow of blood to your heart, it can cause a heart attack. When a clot blocks the flow of blood to your brain, it can cause a stroke.

Very low density lipoprotein (VLDL) carries even more risk than LDL. It is the largest type of lipoprotein.

High density lipoprotein is known as good cholesterol. That's because it carries cholesterol away from the arteries to the liver, where it is broken down and disposed of. While high levels of LDL cholesterol are predictors of future heart problems, the opposite is true of HDL cholesterol. A high level of HDL seems to protect against heart disease and stroke.

Triglycerides are another type of fat that circulate in your blood. A high level of triglycerides can also be a warning sign of future heart disease.

You can't tell when your cholesterol levels are high. High cholesterol won't make you dizzy or tired, and you can't look at someone and say, "Gee, you don't look so good. Your cholesterol levels must be high." The only way to know if your cholesterol is high is to have it checked by a simple blood test.

The National Heart, Lung and Blood Institute recommends you have a cholesterol screening every five years, beginning at age 20. Some experts think you should have it checked more often because cholesterol levels may fluctuate for various reasons.

Before having your cholesterol screened, don't eat anything for 12 hours. It's also important to avoid drinking alcohol or doing any vigorous exercise for 24 hours before the test.

🐝 🐝 🐝

Southern grapes good for the heart

Most traditional Southern cooking isn't known for being heart-healthy. Gravy, fried pork chops, and buttered biscuits and grits may taste great, but they add too much fat to your diet and shoot your cholesterol higher than a Georgia pine.

The South does have at least one healthy food to contribute to the cause of good heart health — a grape known as the muscadine or scuppernong. Southern cooks have long made use of this tough-skinned but tasty fruit by making jams, preserves, juice, wine, and even muscadine hull pies.

Scientists have found that this modest fruit contains substantial amounts of resveratrol, the substance in red wine believed to contribute to a healthy heart. Muscadines are high in fiber and carbohydrates but low in fat and protein. Although the effects of muscadines on humans haven't been studied yet, one animal study found that this little fruit lowered LDL cholesterol and raised HDL cholesterol.

If you don't drink wine but would like to take advantage of the heart-protecting effect of resveratrol, try some muscadine jam on your toast. One serving contains as much resveratrol as 4 ounces of red wine.

🐝 🐝

Defend yourself against the latest bad guy

For years now, LDL has been known as the bad cholesterol. Now research has identified a particularly dangerous and stubborn form of LDL, called lipoprotein(a), or Lp(a). One study found that women with very high Lp(a) levels had almost double the risk of having a heart attack.

The reason Lp(a) is so destructive may be its design. It has an extra strand of sticky protein that regular LDL cholesterol doesn't have. This makes it resemble another substance in your blood that is designed to break up clots. Scientists think this appearance may trick plaque into soaking up the cholesterol instead of the clot buster.

Lp(a) is also very unlikely to respond to conventional cholesterol treatment. So far, the only effective treatments are niacin and estrogen.

Your doctor may not routinely screen for Lp(a). Make sure you ask if it's included in your cholesterol screening.

	Ideal	Near/ Above ideal	Border- line high	High	Very high
Total cholesterol	Less than 200		200-239	240 and above	
LDL cholesterol	Less than 100	100-129	130-159	160-189	190 and above
Triglycerides	Less than 150		150-199	200-499	500 and above

	Low	Average	High
HDL cholesterol	Less than 40	40-60	61 and above

Do-it-yourself cholesterol testing

For about $20, you can buy an at-home testing kit called CholesTrak from your drugstore. You just prick your finger with a device that's included and squeeze two or three drops of blood onto the test strip. You'll get results in about 15 minutes.

CholesTrak is supposed to be as accurate as a professional lab test, but it only measures total cholesterol. If your reading is over 200, you'll still need to make an appointment with your doctor to get a total profile, including HDL, LDL, and triglyceride levels.

{a. {a.

Get the facts about cholesterol-lowering drugs

Your cholesterol was high when you had it checked, so you changed your diet and started exercising. For about 90 percent of the people, these changes are enough to bring cholesterol under control. If your level still hasn't budged after making these lifestyle changes, your doctor may decide to prescribe cholesterol-lowering drugs.

While drugs shouldn't be substituted for a healthy diet and regular exercise, they can help bring your cholesterol levels under control, especially if you have other risk factors for heart disease.

Statins (HMG-CoA reductase inhibitors). These drugs work by blocking an enzyme your body needs to manufacture cholesterol. They are usually your doctor's first choice for treating high cholesterol because they are the most effective at lowering LDL levels. A recent study found that statins reduced the risk of stroke by 29 percent and the risk of death from heart disease by 28 percent. Side effects are rare and usually mild, but a few people may develop liver problems. You should have liver function tests periodically while taking these medications. A recent study found that one statin, atorvastatin (Lipitor), was more effective than others. Other commonly prescribed statins include cerivastatin (Baycol), fluvastatin (Lescol), lovastatin (Mevacor), pravastatin (Pravachol), and simvastatin (Zocor).

Bile acid binding resins. These work by attaching to cholesterol-containing substances in your intestines. Since these drugs are not absorbed by your body, the substances also pass out of your body without being absorbed. Constipation is the most common side effect. Others include abdominal discomfort, flatulence, nausea, and heartburn. These drugs also

interfere with your body's ability to absorb the fat-soluble vitamins — A, D, E, and K. Ask your doctor if you need vitamin
supplements while taking these drugs. Because of their effect
on vitamin K, which is needed for blood clotting, they can
interact with blood-thinning medication. Commonly prescribed bile acid binding resins include cholestyramine
(Questran) and colestipol (Colestid).

Fibrates (fibric acid analogs). These work by reducing
your liver's ability to manufacture cholesterol. Usually, gemfibrozil (Lopid) is more effective than statins at reducing triglycerides, but it's not as effective at lowering LDL cholesterol. Side
effects of gemfibrozil include nausea, flatulence, abdominal
discomfort, bloating, and mild liver problems. Side effects of
clofibrate (Atromid-S) can be more severe. It has been associated with increased risk of gallstones and serious gastrointesti-
nal disease, including liver cancer. Fibrates shouldn't be used in
combination with statins because the risk of muscle tissue disorders is greatly increased.

Nicotinic acid (niacin). Niacin, also known as vitamin
B3, can help increase HDL levels, reduce total and LDL cholesterol, and decrease triglyceride levels by up to 50 percent.
Possible side effects include flushing, itching, abdominal discomfort, and gout. It can also affect your liver. Taking 325 milligrams (mg) of aspirin 30 minutes before taking niacin can
reduce flushing. A chemical cousin of niacin, called inositol
hexanicotinate (IHN), acts as well as, or better than, niacin
without the bothersome side effect of flushing. To lessen
abdominal discomfort, take niacin with meals. Avoid drinking
alcohol or hot beverages right after you take it.

If you want to try niacin to lower your cholesterol or triglycerides, let your doctor know. People with liver problems, diabetes, ulcers, gout, or heart problems should only take niacin
under a doctor's care because it can worsen these conditions.

Pros and cons of cholesterol-lowering drugs

Niacin

Pros
- Lowers LDL and triglycerides
- Raises HDL
- Least expensive cholesterol-lowering drug

Cons
- Highest toxicity risk
- Causes side effects like flushing and itching
- May cause liver and blood sugar problems

Special warnings
- Loss of appetite, nausea, indigestion, or flulike symptoms may be signs of niacin toxicity; call your doctor immediately
- Take only with meals
- Take at least some of your dose at night, when your body makes the most cholesterol
- Time-released niacin may cause more liver problems than regular niacin

Statins

Pros
- Very effective at lowering LDL and good at lowering triglycerides
- HDL may increase
- Can slow down or reverse atherosclerosis

Cons
- Expensive
- Can cause liver or muscle inflammation
- If untreated, inflammation could lead to kidney failure
- May or may not prevent heart attacks

Special warnings
- Liver and muscle enzymes should be checked regularly
- Muscle aches could be a sign of toxicity
- Take at least some of your dose at night, when your body makes the most cholesterol
- Talk to your doctor if you are also taking gemfibrozil (Lopid)

Fibrates

Pros
- Lowers triglycerides
- Raises HDL

Cons
- Expensive
- Not as effective at lowering LDL as statins
- May cause gallstones
- Clofibrate (Atromid) reduces heart attack risk but increases the proportion of heart attacks that are fatal
- Atromid increases cancer risk

Special warnings
- Atromid's negative effects outweigh its positive effects
- Lopid may lower triglycerides but raise LDL
- Call your doctor if you have nausea, abdominal pain, or other symptoms of gallstones

Bile acid binding resins

Pros
- Not absorbed into body, so few problems with liver and blood sugar
- Lowers LDL
- Sometimes raises HDL

Cons:
- Expensive
- May cause abdominal discomfort
- Reduced absorption of vitamins, minerals, or other medicines taken within a few hours of bile acid binding resin drug
- May increase triglycerides

Special warnings
- Reduce stomach upset by taking with wheat bran or Metamucil
- Take one hour before meals
- Reduce the chance of increasing triglycerides by combining with Lopid
- Take other medicines one hour before or four hours after taking a bile acid resin drug

Fats at a glance

Kind of Fat	Sources	Effect on cholesterol levels	Action advice
Saturated (solid at room temperature)	Meats, butter, lard, whole milk, cheese, palm oil, coconut oil, chocolate	Raises both LDL and HDL cholesterol	Limit to no more than 7 percent of calories daily. Eat lean cuts of meat and use low-fat dairy products.
Polyunsaturated (liquid at room temperature)	Vegetable oils: corn, safflower, sunflower, sesame, soybean, cottonseed	Reduces both HDL and LDL cholesterol. Too much may increase cancer risk.	Use oils and soft margarine in moderation, keeping total fat at or below 35 percent of calories per day.
Mono-unsaturated (liquid at room temperature)	Olive oil, peanut oil, canola oil, nuts, avocado	Lowers LDL. HDL stays the same or may be raised in some cases.	Use freely up to 35 percent of total calories per day.
Trans fatty acids (solid at room temperature)	Margarines, vegetable shortenings	Raises LDL. Lowers HDL	Reduce or avoid commercially baked products (breads, cookies, cakes) and fried foods from fast-food restaurants. Look for recipes that offer other options in cooking.

Wipe out cholesterol with hard work

You may think you're working hard to reduce your cholesterol, but if you want an example to follow, take a look at the Mennonites.

Researchers studying a group of Old Order Mennonites, a religious group living in New York state, found that although they ate as much fat and cholesterol as other Americans, their cholesterol levels were much lower.

According to the study, Mennonite men eat about 600 more calories per day on average than most men. However, they are leaner and have an average cholesterol level of 177, compared with 192 for most other men.

The key may be their lifestyle. Most Mennonites work hard on farms, and they don't rely on motorized vehicles for transportation.

If you truly want to lower your cholesterol, take a hint from the Mennonites, and just work a little harder.

High Blood Pressure

~

5 reasons to control high blood pressure

How long would it take you to travel 60,000 miles? That's about how much distance your blood vessels cover. Your heart has to pump hard enough to force your blood through all those veins and arteries. It pumps about 3 ounces of blood with every beat, which adds up to about 2,000 gallons a day.

In performing this monumental task, your heart creates pressure in your blood vessels. Your blood pressure is actually the result of two forces — your heart pushing blood into your blood vessels, and the force of your arteries resisting the flow. Healthy blood vessels are elastic, so they can withstand this force and spring back.

When your blood pressure is too high, your blood is pushing against the walls of your arteries with more force than normal. This condition, also known as hypertension, sounds like something that occurs only if you're hyperactive or tense, but that isn't the case.

Most people with high blood pressure don't even know they have it, yet it affects almost one in four adults. If so many people are walking around with this "silent" condition, you may think it can't be very serious. You couldn't be more wrong.

High blood pressure can affect almost every organ in your body. It can increase your risk of developing aneurysms, loss of vision, memory loss, and these other serious health problems:

- **Atherosclerosis.** Arteriosclerosis (hardening of the arteries) is a natural process of aging in which your arteries become thicker and stiffer. Over time, high blood pressure can speed up the process and make it easier for fatty deposits to stick to your artery walls and create blockages. Atherosclerosis is a form of arteriosclerosis. This means you have cholesterol or other fatty deposits, along with hardening of your arteries.

- **Heart attack.** If your arteries become narrowed by plaque, blood flow is blocked to that portion of the heart muscle. If the blood flow is blocked completely, you could have a heart attack.

- **Enlarged heart.** When you have high blood pressure, your heart has to work harder, which can cause it to become enlarged. Eventually it could stop working properly and cause fluids to back up into your lungs.

- **Kidney damage.** Your kidneys help your body get rid of waste products. High blood pressure can damage the blood vessels that carry blood into your kidneys for cleansing. When this happens, waste products can build up in your blood and become toxic.

- **Stroke.** The damage high blood pressure does to your arteries can lead to a stroke. One type of stroke, called a thrombotic stroke, occurs when a clot blocks a narrow artery. Another type occurs when extremely high blood pressure causes a weakened blood vessel in your brain to rupture. This is called a hemorrhagic stroke.

The best defense against high blood pressure

High blood pressure usually doesn't cause any symptoms, which is why it's called the "silent epidemic." The only way to know for sure if you have it is to have your blood pressure checked regularly.

Blood pressure is usually taken with an arm-pressure cuff, called a sphygmomanometer (sfig-mo-ma-nom-e-ter), which comes from two Greek words that mean pulse measurement. When your doctor or other health care worker takes your blood pressure, it is recorded as two separate numbers, for example, 120/80 (120 over 80).

The first, or top, number refers to systolic pressure, or the pressure that is produced as the heart contracts to pump blood out into the body. The second, or bottom, number refers to diastolic pressure, or the pressure that remains in the blood vessels as the heart relaxes to allow blood to flow into the ventricles, the pumping chambers of the heart.

Both of these numbers are important to your doctor because they give him a great deal of information about the health of your cardiovascular system — your heart, arteries, arterioles, capillaries, and veins.

The systolic pressure is important because it tells the maximum amount of pressure placed on your arteries. The diastolic is equally important, telling the minimum pressure on your arteries. The harder it is for blood to flow through your vessels, the higher both numbers will be.

When someone takes your blood pressure with a standard sphygmomanometer, a cuff containing an inflatable bladder is wrapped around your upper arm, with the middle of the bladder placed directly over your brachial artery, the large artery in your arm.

This bladder is connected to a needle-valved rubber bulb by a piece of rubber tubing. Air is pumped into the cuff by squeezing the rubber bulb. As the bulb is pumped and the bladder begins to fill with air, the pressure in the cuff goes up.

This pressure is shown on the calibrated tube of mercury. The bladder is pumped up until it stops the flow of blood in your arm. Using a stethoscope placed over your brachial artery, the person taking your blood pressure listens to the sound of blood pulsing through the artery. When that pulsing sound stops, the examiner knows the cuff has been pumped up enough to stop blood flow in that artery.

At that point, the examiner turns the valve on the bulb to begin slowly releasing air from the bladder. As the valve is turned and the air begins to escape from the cuff, blood is able to flow through the artery again, and the first pulse sound is heard through the stethoscope.

The sharp tapping or knocking sounds generated by the blood pulsing through the artery are known as Korotkoff sounds. The height of the mercury or the number on the gauge is noted when the first pulse is heard. This is the systolic level.

As the air continues to be released from the cuff, the pulse sounds get stronger, then fade. When they finally fade away, another steady sound is heard. This is the sound of the blood flowing through the veins. The number on the gauge at this point is your diastolic pressure.

Categories for blood pressure levels in adults*
(Age 18 years and older)

| Category | Blood pressure | |
	Systolic (top number)	Diastolic (bottom number)
Normal	Less than 120	Less than 80
Prehypertension	120-139	80-89
Stage 1	140-159	90-99
Stage 2 higher	160 and higher	100 and

*For those not taking medicine for high blood pressure and not having a short-term, serious illness. If you are over 50, and your systolic pressure (the top number) is more than 140, your doctor should begin treating you for high blood pressure — regardless of your diastolic pressure (the bottom number).

Simple test helps determine artery health

You can find out more about the condition of your arteries by having your doctor take an additional blood pressure reading around your ankle.

You divide your ankle reading by your arm reading, and if your number is .90 or lower, that's a red flag you may be headed for trouble. One study found that people with an ankle/arm index of .80 or lower were five times as likely to die of heart disease.

A low ankle/arm index indicates that you may have blocked arteries in your legs. Some people with leg-vessel blockage will have pain when they walk, but many people have no symptoms. Adding the ankle reading to your usual checkup may be the best way for you to avoid heart problems later.

7 successful strategies for lowering blood pressure

The first step in protecting your heart and arteries is having your blood pressure measured. If it's high, it's time to do something about it. There's not much you can do about your age or family history of high blood pressure, but most risk factors are within your control. Here are some natural strategies to help lower your blood pressure:

- **Lose weight.** If you're overweight, this may be the most helpful thing you can do for your blood pressure and your overall health. Weight loss significantly reduces blood pressure in most people with high blood pressure.

- **Limit your salt intake.** Not everyone will benefit from limiting their salt intake. Some people are not "salt sensitive." But if you are, eating less salt can help lower your blood pressure.

- **Get enough calcium, magnesium, and potassium.** These minerals play an important role in maintaining blood pressure levels.

- **Watch your fat and cholesterol.** Try to limit your intake of saturated fat and foods high in cholesterol.

- **Exercise.** Regular exercise alone can help lower your blood pressure. If you also lose weight, you'll lower it even more.

- **Limit your alcohol.** Too much alcohol can increase your blood pressure. Many people have high blood pressure solely because they drink too much alcohol. Daily intake should be no more than 24 ounces of beer, 8 ounces of wine, or 2 ounces of liquor.

- **Stop smoking.** People with high blood pressure who smoke are three to five times more likely to die from heart disease than nonsmokers.

The latest scoop on blood pressure drugs

Because some high blood pressure medications have gotten a lot of negative publicity, you may be wondering if the cure isn't worse than the disease.

While you should do all you can to lower your blood pressure naturally, some people need medication to lower their blood pressure and prevent complications. These types of drugs are commonly prescribed.

Calcium channel blockers. These drugs work by affecting the movement of calcium into the cells of your heart and blood vessels. They relax your blood vessels and increase the blood and oxygen supply to your heart.

Controversy surrounds the use of calcium channel blockers, mostly the short-acting ones. A recent study found that postmenopausal women who took calcium channel blockers were twice as likely to develop breast cancer as other women. Other studies have found an increase in deaths and heart attacks among people taking short-acting nifedipine, a calcium channel blocker. The safety of longer-acting calcium channel blockers is also being questioned and studied. Other drugs may be safer for many people now taking calcium channel blockers.

The National Heart, Lung, and Blood Institute recommends to doctors that "short-acting nifedipine should be used with great caution (if at all), especially at higher doses in the treatment of hypertension (high blood pressure), angina, and MI (myocardial infarction)." The American Heart Association cautions people who are already taking this drug not to suddenly stop taking it without consulting their doctors.

ACE inhibitors. ACE stands for angiotensin converting enzyme. ACE inhibitors work by blocking a chemical called angiotensin in your body that causes blood vessels to tighten. As a result, ACE inhibitors relax your blood vessels. This lowers your blood pressure and increases the supply of blood and oxygen to your heart. A recent study found that ACE inhibitors also improved people's chances of surviving after a heart attack.

Some ACE inhibitors may increase potassium levels. When those drugs are combined with potassium-sparing diuretics, the situation could be life-threatening. Elderly people, diabetics, and people with kidney problems are at the highest risk.

Dizziness, headache, fatigue, and coughing are side effects of ACE inhibitors. Loss of taste might occur with the use of captopril.

Diuretics. Diuretics work on your kidneys to increase urination and get rid of excess fluid. They are probably the most commonly recommended high blood pressure medication — and the most inexpensive.

One problem with diuretics is that you may be flushing too many minerals out with your urine, including potassium, which is important for your heart's health. Sometimes potassium supplements are recommended if you are taking diuretics, or your doctor may prescribe a potassium-sparing diuretic.

Loop diuretics are another type of diuretic. They are so-named because they work in a part of the kidney called the Loop of Henle. This makes them more effective.

Beta blockers. These drugs lower blood pressure by blocking certain actions of your sympathetic nervous system. They expand blood vessel walls and slow down the contractions of your heart.

Commonly prescribed blood pressure medications

ACE inhibitors	benazepril (Lotensin), captopril (Capoten), enalapril (Vasotec), fosinopril (Monopril), lisinopril (Prinivil, Zestril), quinapril (Accupril), ramipril (Altace)
Calcium channel blockers	amlodipine (Norvasc), diltiazem (Cardizem), felodipine (Plendil), isradipine (DynaCirc), nicardipine (Cardene), nifedipine (Adalat, Procardia), verapamil (Calan, Isoptin, Verelan)
Beta blockers	acebutolol (Sectral), atenolol (Tenormin), betaxolol (Kerlone), carteolol (Cartrol), propranolol (Inderal), metoprolol (Lopressor), nadolol (Corgard)

Commonly prescribed diuretics

Thiazides and related diuretics	chlorothiazide (Diuril), chlorthalidone (Thalitone), hydrochlorothiazide (Esidrix, HydroDIURIL, Oretic), hydroflumethiazide (Diucardin), methyclothiazide (Enduron), metolazone (Mykrox, Zaroxolyn)
Loop diuretics	bumetanide (Bumex), ethacrynic acid (Edecrin), furosemide (Lasix)
Potassium-sparing diuretics	amiloride (Midamor), spironolactone (Aldactone), triamterene (Dyrenium)
Combination diuretics	amiloride and hydrochlorothiazide (Moduretic), spironolactone and hydrochlorothiazide (Aldactazide), triamterene and hydrochlorothiazide (Dyazide)

The dangers of prescription drugs

A recent study showed that more than 2 million Americans become ill every year because of reactions to properly prescribed drugs. More than 100,000 people die from these reactions.

The older you become, the less efficient your liver and kidneys are at eliminating drugs from your bloodstream. That means drugs stay in your body longer and build up to higher levels than they would in the body of a younger person.

Older people should ask if there are any side effects that may be more dangerous to them, such as dizziness that may cause falls, drowsiness that may make driving dangerous, and mental confusion that may affect memory. Be sure to note any side effects you experience, no matter how minor they seem.

If you experience side effects, your doctor may decide to change the dose, try another drug, stop the medication, or decide the benefits of the drug outweigh the bad effects you are feeling. You should never make that decision for yourself. Just as you should never take a drug without your doctor's consent, you should never stop taking medication without consulting him.

🐞 🐞 🐞

Don't get burned — follow doctor's advice

If you're having misgivings about your blood pressure medication, talk with your doctor, but don't stop taking them without your doctor's approval.

A recent study found that people who stop taking their blood pressure medication were almost five times as likely to suffer a deadly type of stroke.

The study also found that smokers were over six times as likely to have this kind of stroke — called a hemorrhagic or bleeding stroke.

So if you smoke, stop. But if your doctor has prescribed blood pressure medication for you, don't stop ... at least not without his permission.

🐞 🐞

High blood pressure drugs that steal sexual desire

Drug	Common brand names
Methyldopa	Aldoclor, Aldomet
Propranolol hydrochloride	Inderal, Inderide
Guanethidine monosulfate	Esimil, Ismelin
Reserpine	Diupres, Hydropres
Prazosin hydrochloride	Minipress, Minizide
Clonidine	Catapres-TTS

Beware of the 'grapefruit effect'

If you're taking medicine for your high blood pressure, be careful what you wash it down with. Grapefruit juice in the morning may be nutritious and delicious, but it could cause your blood pressure drug to build up to toxic levels in your body.

The "grapefruit effect" on drugs was discovered accidentally by researchers several years ago when they gave volunteers grapefruit juice to hide the taste of a medication. They found out that when the medicine was taken with grapefruit juice, it multiplied the amount of the medication in the blood.

Later studies found that grapefruit contains a substance that blocks the effects of an enzyme, which helps break down certain types of drugs in your body. Instead of being metabolized, the drugs continue to circulate in your body and accumulate.

Although the grapefruit effect could help make some drugs more effective, consider the American Heart Association's recommendation — don't drink grapefruit juice about the same time as taking calcium channel blockers.

Other drugs that may be affected by grapefruit juice include some types of sleeping pills, antihistamines, and cyclosporine. Ask your doctor or pharmacist if grapefruit juice will affect your medication.

Licorice alert

Those who like to snack on licorice candy every day may be left with a bad taste in their mouths after hearing this news: Licorice can raise your blood pressure. Adults who eat large quantities of real licorice, not artificially flavored, every day run a higher than normal risk of developing high blood pressure and heart disease.

Apparently, licorice or licorice extract causes your body to retain sodium and fluids and lose potassium, which raises blood pressure and puts a strain on your heart.

Researchers recommend that licorice lovers with high blood pressure cut way back on their treat and eat it only on special occasions.

Of course, most licorice sold in the United States is now made with artificial flavoring, usually anise oil, so it's safe for you to eat. The ingredient you want to avoid is glycyrrhizic acid. This ingredient is highly concentrated in some licorice candies and in some laxatives and tobacco products.

Hot tubs — what you should know before jumping in

You probably know that exercise and stress can make your blood pressure rise. But did you know that relaxing in a steamy sauna or hot tub can also make it rise?

If you have high blood pressure, you don't have to give up your dips in the hot tub. It only makes your blood pressure rise about as much as a brisk walk. However, if you have any symptoms, like shortness of breath or chest pain, you might want to skip the soak and call your doctor.

You should also avoid drinking alcohol before or during your sauna. And be aware that moving back and forth between cold water, like a swimming pool, and a hot tub or sauna can shoot your blood pressure up even higher.

Alcohol

Moderation is the key to heart health

If you don't drink alcohol, doctors are not telling you to start. There are several serious health reasons why you should not drink, such as liver disease, pancreatitis, high blood pressure, congestive heart failure, or a history of alcoholism. And keep in mind that certain medications interact with alcohol and could cause serious side effects. No amount of heart benefit from alcohol could outweigh the risks you might be taking under these conditions.

However, if you drink already, the key word here is "moderation." You may find several definitions of moderate drinking, but most experts agree that "one drink" equals a 12-ounce bottle of beer, a 4-ounce glass of wine, or a 1 1/2-ounce shot of 80-proof spirits. Consuming one or two of these drinks a day is usually considered moderate drinking.

Studies have shown that consuming larger amounts of alcohol will actually damage your heart muscle and possibly the tissues in your arteries. Long-time alcoholics suffer most from this damage, which is called alcoholic cardiomyopathy.

To keep it all in perspective, picture a graph that looks like the letter "J." If you drink absolutely no alcohol, your risk of heart disease places you on the tip of the small hook — not too high a danger, but not the lowest, either. By taking one to two alcoholic drinks a day, you travel down the "J" to its base point, actually decreasing your risk. The more alcohol you consume each day, the further up the long side of the "J" you go, increasing your risk of heart disease, and all other causes of death, along the way.

For more information about alcohol and heart health, see the *Grapes and red wine* chapter.

Researchers continue to study alcohol's effects

The word ethanol may conjure up images of car motors and gas tanks, but if you know your chemistry, you'll recognize it as the intoxicating ingredient in liquor, wine, and beer. Now scientists are wondering if this is really the secret to alcohol's beneficial effect on heart disease, since ethanol has been proven to actually increase HDL cholesterol. And a higher HDL level means a lower risk of heart disease.

In addition, ethanol may affect the way your blood clots, either by causing it to clot less or by helping it break up clots when they do form. A drink with dinner might help protect your arteries even into the following day.

To find out if this is true, researchers, headed by Dr. Eric Rimm of Harvard's Department of Nutrition, reviewed studies of alcohol and the risk of coronary heart disease dating back to 1965. They found it isn't just wine that has been linked with heart-healthy benefits. Beer and other liquors seem to be just as beneficial.

The American Cancer Society conducted its own study of almost half a million people, ranging in age from 30 to 104. What they found confirms Rimm's analysis. It's not so much what you drink, but how much. If people would drink small amounts over a longer period of time, they would experience more health benefits and less injury from alcohol.

Alcohol's effects on two killer heart conditions

Two recent studies out of Boston's Brigham and Women's Hospital show that the risk of angina and heart attack are decreased by moderate drinking. According to the studies, men taking two or more alcoholic drinks per day lowered their risk of developing angina by more than half and their risk of heart attack by almost half. Also, men who had already suffered either a heart attack or stroke and had one or two alcoholic drinks a day reduced their risk of a second heart attack by almost a third.

If you have high blood pressure, most doctors will tell you not to drink alcohol because it can cause your blood pressure to go even higher. In fact, one study revealed that men who drank the most alcohol had the highest incidence of high blood pressure. However, research has proven that moderate drinkers have either similar or lower blood pressure readings than nondrinkers.

If you do drink and need to watch your blood pressure, remember moderation, and be sure to eat plenty of fresh fruits and vegetables, which are good sources of potassium and calcium. These two minerals work together to counteract the bad effects of alcohol and to keep your blood pressure from shooting through the roof.

To boost your potassium and calcium intake, give some of these foods a try.

Potassium	potatoes, squash, raisins, dried apricots, avocados
Calcium	rhubarb, bok choy, spinach, legumes, dried figs

Women more susceptible to damage than men

While many women have claimed for years that they are the more sensitive sex, they probably didn't have muscle sensitivity in mind. Unfortunately, science has proven this to be the case. Researchers at the University of Barcelona, Spain, found that women's hearts were more susceptible to muscle damage from alcohol than men's — even when they drank much less.

When deciding whether or not to drink, you must weigh this information against the fact that women who drink any amount of alcohol at all decrease their risk of heart disease by 20 percent, compared to women who abstain. Having one-half to two drinks a day reduces heart disease risk by almost 40 percent.

However, if you throw hormone replacement therapy and the risk of breast cancer into the equation, things become more confusing.

Some studies prove that regular alcohol use can raise estrogen levels. This keeps your bones dense and strong and helps in the fight against osteoporosis. However, if you take estrogen and have the equivalent of about one drink every day, you increase your risk of developing breast cancer.

Some experts believe that simply reducing the amount of alcohol you drink can offset this risk. It wouldn't hurt to eat more vegetables like cabbage, broccoli, and turnips, either.

People at risk reap the most benefits

According to Dr. Vincent M. Figueredo, assistant professor of medicine at the University of California, San Francisco, School of Medicine, those who can benefit the most from moderate, regular alcohol use are:

- men over 40 at high risk of heart disease
- premenopausal women at high risk of heart disease but with no family history of breast cancer
- postmenopausal women

The majority of deaths from alcohol abuse occur in young people, while the majority of lives saved by alcohol are in the preceding three categories. The challenge health professionals face is getting the message of moderate drinking out to those with the most to gain.

Alcohol and medication — a bad idea

You may think washing down your blood pressure medicine with a little glass of wine won't hurt a thing. After all, you've heard that red wine is supposed to be beneficial for your heart. But mixing alcohol with any drug, either prescription or over-the-counter, could be a dangerous mistake.

Many older people take medicine, and some take several different kinds for different ailments. The side effects of consuming alcohol with sedatives, antidepressants, anticoagulants, or prescription drugs for high blood pressure include dangerous bleeding, changes in blood pressure, and serious stomach irritation. It only takes a small amount of alcohol to cause these reactions, especially in elderly people.

Taking over-the-counter NSAIDs such as aspirin and ibuprofen can cause bleeding in your stomach. If you take them with alcohol, you're four times as likely to have severe stomach bleeding. The pain reliever acetaminophen, when taken in excess by someone who consumes three or more alcoholic drinks a day, may cause serious liver damage.

Alexander Technique

Take control of your health

There are many roads to better health. One of them involves training your mind and body to work together for perfect coordination and movement. Better heart health might start with something as simple as the way your head, neck, and back are balanced.

Frederick Matthias Alexander was a Shakespearean actor who lived around the turn of the 20th century. When he developed chronic laryngitis, doctors said there was little besides surgery that could help.

Alexander, however, was determined to help himself. He began studying and changing his own body movements and muscle tension in an effort to reduce the strain on his neck and vocal chords. In the process, he discovered he had been abusing his voice, as well as his entire body. When he began to change the way he moved, his voice returned and his overall health improved.

The method he developed and began teaching to others, called the Alexander Technique, is a way of using your body. Through his approach, you learn how to get rid of harmful tension, stress, strain, pain, fatigue, and depression. These are often hidden causes of all kinds of physical problems, including high blood pressure.

It's not an exercise program but a relearning of habits, both physical and mental. You relax your body; improve your breathing, posture, and balance; and calm your mind. You learn how to use your muscles in a more efficient way so you can cope better with daily life. You'll discover the best way to do all kinds of everyday activities, like lie down, get up, stand, walk, run, reach, lift, climb, and drive.

If you want to take responsibility for your own health and well-being, try the Alexander Technique.

Although you can find books on the philosophy and fundamentals of the Alexander Technique at your local bookstore or library, you'll need a teacher in order to fully understand and master this technique.

For help finding instruction in the United States, contact:
American Society for the Alexander Technique (AMSAT)
P.O. Box 60008
Florence, MA 01062
800-473-0620

In Canada:
Canadian Society of Teachers of the Alexander Technique (CANSTAT)
RPO 984 West Broadway
P.O. Box 53568
Vancouver, BC
Canada, V5Z 1K0
877-598-8879

Anger Arresters

Chill out ... and lower your risk of heart disease

Remember the part of the movie where a character, usually an older, overweight man, has an angry outburst so severe he clutches his chest, has a heart attack, and dies? Unfortunately, this scene is more fact than fiction. Anger can kill.

In the 1960s, when the first studies on type A personality were done, researchers found scientific evidence that being aggressive, driven, competitive, and time-pressured can physically damage your heart. Medical studies in recent years have shown that the most damaging aspects of a type A personality are anger and hostility.

Angry people, especially men, have a higher risk of heart problems. A personality profile that includes irritability, getting angry easily, and frequent outbursts may double or even triple your risk of heart disease, including angina and heart attack. Getting angry even raises your cholesterol level.

When you become angry, your heart rate increases and your blood pressure goes up. At the same time, your heart needs more oxygen to function at its faster speed. Arteries already narrowed from a buildup of plaque may constrict to become even narrower, so blood has more trouble flowing through them. While this is going on, the platelets in your blood clot more easily, possibly narrowing your arteries further or even causing a blockage. This could lead to a heart attack or stroke.

It would be easy to simply say, "Don't ever lose your temper or feel hostile again." But that's not a real possibility for most people. However, you can learn ways to deal with your anger to protect your heart from damage and keep yourself on a more even keel.

Manage your anger to protect your heart

If you think you should just hold an explosive case of anger in check, think again. Researchers have discovered a new type of personality to describe the kind of person who holds his emotions inside — type D. Instead of being openly aggressive and hostile like a type A personality, someone with a type D personality is just as angry and hostile, but he covers it up and holds on to the anger. If you are a type-D person who simply swallows emotional distress like a bitter pill, you might want to change your ways. If you have heart disease, your chances of death are four times higher than people who aren't type D.

Letting your anger seethe like a simmering pot will eventually cause your body to release stress hormones. These hormones cause your blood pressure to go up and your arteries to narrow. It also weakens your immune system so you're more open to attack by passing viruses and bacteria.

Anger kept at a slow boil can show up in other physical problems, too, including overeating and alcohol abuse. These habits can do more harm to your heart.

But you don't have to hold your anger inside all the time. And you don't have to wait until you finally explode, sometimes at a completely innocent person, and feel horribly guilty afterward.

With practice, anger can be managed and controlled. Having a plan to manage your anger gives you the tools you need to defuse a heart-hurting situation. Get familiar with this list and use whichever tools work best for you. Here are the steps to take immediately when you feel anger rising.

- **Take deep breaths.** You'll help get much-needed oxygen to your racing heart and help yourself calm down and relax. That old saying about counting to 10 is good advice, too. Just count slowly and think calm thoughts.

- **Express it, then forget it.** If you express your anger, do so in a constructive way. Wait until you are calm and can say what you need to without exploding. State clearly why you are angry, but try not to accuse others if you can help it. You might be able to bring about positive change in a situation. But even if nothing changes, express yourself, then let it go. No matter how important an issue seems to you at the time, letting it drop is more important for your heart's health than holding on to it and fuming inside.

- **Talk it out.** Talking with a loved one or close friend about an issue that is angering you will usually help you get a clearer perspective. You may find that the issue isn't worth exploring any further, or you may come up with a good plan of attack to solve the problem.

- **Give the other guy a break.** Always competing, getting angry if you're not the first in line, and passing everyone on the highway is a way of life for some people. This anger and stress can hurt your heart. Try letting go and letting the other guy win sometimes. You may find that once you stop competing, the other person will stop and act more gracious, too.

The following steps for coping with anger are ones to take over the long haul. Even though you may not get immediate results, stick with them, and you should see dramatic improvements in your ability to handle anger.

- **Exercise.** Along with strengthening your heart and lowering your blood pressure, regular exercise reduces stress and gives you a feeling of well-being. If you're feeling angry, a long walk may be just the thing to help you replace bad feelings with good ones. Schedule time to exercise at least three days a week for 20 minutes or longer at a stretch.

- **Help others.** If you're angry much of the time, it's probably because you are focusing on yourself and your feelings. Try doing some volunteer work or helping out a neighbor or friend who could use a hand. Giving of yourself helps you get a better focus on the rest of the world.

- **Work it off.** If you feel like striking out at someone, try putting your energy in another direction. Clean out a closet, do some weeding in your garden, or cook a healthy gourmet meal. You can accomplish something positive, work off some of your angry energy, and give yourself a little time and distance to cool off.

- **Escape.** Sometimes a short "mental vacation" is just what you need to give you some distance and perspective on the situation you're reacting to. Read a book, watch a pleasant movie, or lose yourself in your favorite hobby. Then you can go back to working on the anger-producing problem with a calmer attitude.

- **Meditate.** Learning to meditate can help you put events in your life in better perspective. Instead of getting angry about the countless little things that can go wrong in a day, choose to let go of them so anger never arises at all. Save your anger for the things that really matter and use it to spur you into action.

◆ **Avoid the issue.** Perhaps the smartest way to deal with anger is to avoid the situations you know will cause it. If shopping in crowded stores infuriates you, shop on Tuesday nights when the fewest people are out, instead of on Saturdays or the day after Thanksgiving. If traffic makes you crazy, arrange to go in to work earlier or later than the rush hour, and leave at an off time, too. If discussing politics with your brother-in-law always leads to a heated argument, don't be drawn into a conversation. You can choose to live your life in ways that lead to a calmer, happier attitude and a healthier heart.

🐜 🐜 🐜

The perfect antidote for stress

Laughter has been called jogging for your internal organs. That may explain why your sides hurt when you laugh really hard.

Besides having a positive effect on your mind, laughter is good for your body. When you laugh, you breathe deeper, which puts more oxygen in your bloodstream, and your diaphragm contracts and relaxes. Your heart rate and blood pressure also increase when you laugh, like it does when you exercise. However, after laughing, your heart rate and blood pressure decrease to lower levels than before you laughed.

Stress can raise your blood pressure and increase your risk of heart attack or stroke. Humor and laughter can counteract the ill effects of daily stress on your body. Research finds that laughter lowers levels of cortisol, a stress hormone, and increases the number and activity of immune system cells.

If you're going to be a couch potato and watch television instead of exercising, at least put in a good comedy. You'll get an internal workout and maybe afterward you'll be inspired to go jogging.

🐜 🐜

Apples

An apple a day just might keep the doctor away

If you're looking for a convenient, easy-to-carry snack packed with vitamins and minerals, complex carbohydrates, healthy fiber, and a delicious burst of flavor, try the original health food — an apple. The humble apple's sweet crunch packs a powerhouse of nutrients your body needs to fight heart disease, no matter how old you are or what physical condition you're in. The benefits of eating apples stack up in three main categories: food value, fiber, and flavonoids — natural chemicals found in some foods that protect your arteries from cholesterol.

The modestly priced apple is an excellent food value for your dollar. One medium apple, eaten with the skin on, has 81 calories, including 21 grams of complex carbohydrates for steady energy. It contains almost 8 milligrams (mg) of vitamin C, or about 10 percent of the amount you need every day for a host of healthy functions, including giving your immune system a boost.

Apples are a very low-fat food, and in case you're watching your salt intake, apples are sodium-free.

This round, shiny fruit contains two important minerals — magnesium and potassium — necessary for the functioning of a healthy heart. Eating foods rich in magnesium results in lower blood pressure, according to studies by the Harvard School of Public Health. And potassium plays a vital role in lowering blood pressure and keeping your heartbeat steady and regular.

The apple is a champion when it comes to providing fiber in your diet. It contains plenty of heart-healthy soluble fiber to fight cholesterol in your body. A ripe, unpeeled medium apple has 4 to 5 grams of fiber, an admirable score. The best way to eat an apple is with the skin on, but even if you feel compelled to peel, it will still give you up to 2.5 grams of soluble fiber. Eating a fiber-rich snack makes you feel full longer, so if you are watching your weight as part of a defense against heart disease, make apples part of your diet every day.

But the best reason to eat your daily apple may be this: A recent medical study in England found that people who eat plenty of fresh fruit every day have a lower risk of death from heart disease and stroke and a lower death rate from all causes. This crunchy, sweet delight is not only a perfect snack but a lifesaver as well.

Fiber gives cholesterol the brush-off

The soluble fiber found in ripe apples is called pectin. This substance is used to thicken fruit for making jams and jellies. In the body, pectin absorbs water in your stomach and intestines to form a thick gel. This gel keeps your bowels moving as they should, counteracting constipation and diverticular disease. It also helps flush out the toxins that may cause colon cancer when they stay in your body too long.

Pectin helps your heart by lowering the level of cholesterol in your blood, possibly preventing heart disease. A French medical study found that eating two apples a day can lower your cholesterol by as much as 10 to 30 percent — a big pay-off for simply choosing a healthy snack. A recent study at a Minnesota university found additional evidence of pectin's ability to reduce blood cholesterol levels, even in people already on low-fat diets.

When excessive LDL cholesterol stays in your body, it can build up in your arteries, forming hard plaque that slows down blood flow. This can lead to high blood pressure and blockages, which can cause heart attacks and strokes. Eating plenty of soluble fiber in the form of pectin can help short-circuit this damaging process called atherosclerosis.

Pectin works against atherosclerosis in two ways. First, it appears to bind with harmful LDL cholesterol and carry it out of your body. Second, it seems to affect the actual clotting mechanism of blood.

In your body, a blood protein called fibrinogen converts to fibrin, the main building block of a blood clot. A recent medical study in South Africa found that pectin not only lowers overall cholesterol and LDL cholesterol in your blood, but it also affects the actual structure of fibrin in your body. By weakening the structure of the fibrin, the blood clots may become weaker and less troublesome when they are forming in an artery. This gives a head start to your body's own clot-busting system so it can prevent clogged arteries and their dangerous consequences.

Focus on flavonoids to fight heart disease

Antioxidants are substances that do battle in your body against free radicals, the roving molecules thought to be behind much of the damage that illness and aging cause. Flavonoids, found in high concentrations in apples, are compounds that act as antioxidants to fight against the build up of LDL cholesterol in your arteries. This means eating flavonoid-rich apples may lower your risk of heart disease, according to recent research.

Dutch doctors tested 805 men over the age of 65 to see what effect their intake of foods containing flavonoids had on their risk of heart disease. Men who consumed the most flavonoids in the form of tea, apples, and onions had a significantly lower risk of heart disease than those who didn't consume foods high in flavonoids. A follow-up study in Finland reinforced these results — another healthy heart claim for apples.

8 ways to reap the benefits of apples

Now that you know how good apples are for your heart, you'll want to enjoy them to the fullest every day. Here are some tips for getting the most from your apples:

- **Leave the skin on.** Most of the flavonoids in an apple are concentrated in the skin, so don't peel it away.

- **Keep it cool.** Apples will generally keep fresher and longer if you store them in the refrigerator than if you keep them out on the kitchen counter.

- **Substitute with sauce.** Applesauce makes a wonderful fat substitute in sweet baked goods, adding nutrition and fiber while it reduces calories and fat grams. Just replace the oil in the recipe with an equal amount of unsweetened applesauce.

- **Serve as a snack.** All ripe apples are good for eating in their natural state, but some are even better than others. The popular Red Delicious apples are wonderful for munching raw, although they don't hold up well for cooking or baking.

- **Bake an apple pie.** The best apples for pies are ones that remain slightly firm after they're cooked. These include Northern Spy, Granny Smith, McIntosh, Empire, Idared, Jonagold, Newtown Pippin, and Gala.

- **Serve in a salad.** For salads, the apples that hold up best are Red Delicious, Fuji, Winesap, and Cortland, a variety that doesn't turn brown quickly when it's exposed to air.

- **Sauce it.** If you want to make your own applesauce, your best bets are Granny Smith, McIntosh, Rome Beauty, Empire, Idared, and Jonagold.

- **Freeze freely.** If you want to use apples in a dish you plan to freeze, the best varieties to use are Golden Delicious, Granny Smith, Rome Beauty, and Winesap.

French Apple Clafouti

You may use Granny Smith or Rome apples for this recipe.
You can also try ripe pears, peaches, or plums.

4 cups (4 medium to large) apples, sliced and peeled
1 1/2 cups whole milk
4 eggs
1/2 cup all-purpose flour, sifted
1/4 cup sugar
1 1/2 teaspoons pure vanilla extract
1/2 teaspoon ground cinnamon

Preheat oven to 350 degrees F. Prepare a deep 10-inch pie plate with butter-flavored nonstick cooking spray, or use a nonstick pie plate. Arrange apple slices evenly in pie plate.

Use a blender or food processor to combine milk and eggs. Add remaining ingredients; blend 5 seconds. Scrape down sides of blender with a spatula; blend until ingredients are mixed together, about 30 seconds. A bowl and whisk can be used to prepare batter by hand.

Spread batter over apples. Bake 1 hour or until custard forms and cake tests done by inserting a toothpick that comes out clean. Serve warm or at room temperature.

Makes 8 servings

Per serving: 144 Calories; 4g Fat (2g from saturated fat) (24% calories from fat); 5g Protein; 23g Carbohydrate; 97mg Cholesterol; 49mg Sodium

Reprinted with permission from The Art of Cooking for the Diabetic by Mary Abbott Hess, 1996

Orange-Yogurt Dip for Fresh Fruit

1 carton (8 ounces) low-fat plain yogurt
2 tablespoons honey
grated peel of 1/2 orange
2 oranges, peeled, segmented
1 medium apple, unpeeled, sliced*
1 medium banana, peeled, cut into chunks*

In small bowl, combine yogurt, honey, and orange peel. Serve as a dip with oranges, apple and banana.

*Sprinkle cut apple and banana with a small amount of orange or lemon juice to prevent fruit from darkening.

Makes 4 servings

Per serving: 130 Calories; 1g Fat (0.6g from saturated fat) (7% calories from fat); 4g Protein; 32g Carbohydrate; 3mg Cholesterol; 42mg Sodium

This is an official 5 A Day Recipe.
This recipe is provided by Sunkist Growers, Inc.

Aromatherapy

Ancient therapy enhances health and well-being

Aromatherapy is an age-old method of using the scents from plants, herbs, and flowers to heal both the mind and the body. As far back as 2,000 B.C., incense, perfumes, and fragrant ointments were used in religious ceremonies and to heal the sick. Today, modern science is beginning to acknowledge what many people have known all along — aromas can have a tremendous impact on emotional and physical health.

From aniseed to ylang ylang, essential oils are the basis of aromatherapy, an alternative method of healing. These oils are carefully extracted from almost any part of an aromatic plant. They are then distilled and bottled, much like the juice from a grape is extracted to make wine. Since these essential oils are very concentrated, you'll probably have to dilute them with water or a base oil, or mix them with some other material. Follow the instructions carefully. Many essential oils can irritate your skin or tissues if you use them full-strength, and some could even be dangerous.

There are a number of ways to use essential oils.

+ Add them to your bath for relaxation or healing.

- Use them to increase the benefits of massage.

- Inhale them straight from the bottle.

- Use a diffuser, vaporizer, candles, aroma lamps, or pot-pourri burners.

- Spray them in your home, office, or bedroom.

- Make a compress.

Not only can they perk you up or calm you down, some can even help heal many common illnesses by fighting bacteria, viruses, and fungi. Their powerful scents can also affect your emotions.

If they are inhaled, the vapors are absorbed through your lungs into your bloodstream where they are distributed throughout your body. In a massage, the pores of your skin allow the oils to seep in and, in small amounts, make their way into your bloodstream to affect your nervous system and other parts of your body.

Since the art and science of aromatherapy can be a bit complicated, get some professional instruction before you buy or use essential oils. You'll be able to find many books on the subject at your library or local bookstore. Most herb shops carry everything you need to get started.

Learn the heart-saving essentials of essential oils

The next time you're cooking dinner, lean over the pot and take a big whiff. Simply by smelling aromatic herbs like garlic, onion, cayenne, and ginger, you'll be improving circulation, making your blood vessels more elastic, and helping to prevent blood clots.

Aromatherapy can't completely replace medicine or your doctor's care — at least not yet. Some animal studies have shown that inhaling the essential oils of lavender, mint, and basil reduces the amount of cholesterol and plaque build-up in the aorta, a main artery.

Aromatherapy also helps your body deal with stress. Vapors in the essential oils trigger a specific part of your brain to release chemicals, such as serotonin, into your nervous system. The chemicals do their job of calming you or bringing on sleep. When your grandmother sprinkled lavender on her bed linens, she was not just making them smell good, she was helping everyone sleep better.

Experts agree that anxiety and disturbed sleep are two conditions that can make your heart problems worse. Many hospitals have realized this and are now using aromatherapy to reduce stress and encourage good sleep patterns in their patients.

9 scent-sational ways to improve heart health

Researchers continue to study the action of essential oils on the body. Their studies have produced a wealth of information about some common, and not-so-common, aromatic plants.

Camphor. You'd recognize camphor anywhere by its sharp, pungent fragrance, but did you know camphor oil is only taken from the wood of trees over 50 years old? Brown and yellow camphor are toxic, so only white camphor is used in aromatherapy. It stimulates the heart and circulation and may raise low blood pressure.

Clary sage. This special variety of sage has been used for centuries to flavor wines, but oddly enough, you shouldn't use the oil if you are drinking alcohol because it tends to exaggerate the effects. Clary sage oil may lower blood pressure.

Hyssop. Hyssop can be found in everything from soaps and sauces to liqueurs, but this pretty shrub also has a variety of medicinal uses. It is used to help regulate blood pressure.

Juniper. You may have several junipers in your yard but never thought of the scent as heart-saving. Juniper oil acts as a sedative, soothing nerves and reducing anxiety. It also helps stimulate circulation.

Lavender. Lavender is one of the most well-known and versatile herbs. You may want to plant a few near your house just to enjoy its fragrance and beautiful flowers. The scent calms your heart, soothes and relieves stress, and lowers high blood pressure.

Marjoram. This may be one herb you'd only think to find in the kitchen, but marjoram can pull it's weight in aromatherapy, too. It lowers high blood pressure, expands the arteries, relieves anxiety, and brings on restful sleep.

Melissa. This herb may be more commonly known as bee balm for its use in treating bee stings, or lemon balm for its delightful lemony fragrance. It slows breathing and heart rate and lowers blood pressure. It can also relax heart muscle spasms and relieve overstimulation of the heart.

Orange blossom. Orange blossoms were traditionally used in bridal bouquets to calm nervous brides. Today, the orange blossom scent is still used to relieve insomnia, anxiety, and depression. It relaxes the heart muscle and reduces the power of its contractions, which makes it useful in the treatment of palpitations.

Rosemary. This silvery-green bush is a favorite of herb gardeners worldwide. The oil is useful for treating nervous heart disorders, such as palpitations. It also helps lower high cholesterol levels.

Artichokes

Funny-looking vegetable lowers cholesterol

Don't let this prickly, unusual-looking vegetable intimidate you. If you've never cooked or eaten an artichoke, now is the time to try this vitamin-packed, heart-healthy vegetable.

You can buy whole, fresh artichokes or hearts and crowns that are canned or frozen. The whole artichoke is fun and easy to eat. What you buy in the store is actually the flower bud of the artichoke plant, which has been harvested by hand. When you get your artichoke home, simply wash it, cut off the stem, and pull off the outer layer of petals.

Usually, whole artichokes are either steamed or boiled, but don't forget your microwave. If you cook it in a bit of water, lemon juice, and vegetable oil, you may find the flavor so good you don't need a sauce.

After cooking, simply pull the petals off, one by one, and eat the soft lining. Eventually, you'll get to the heart, which is entirely edible and has a great nutty flavor. Because of their flavor and nutrients, artichoke hearts are becoming increasingly popular in stir-fries, pasta dishes, and casseroles.

One medium-sized artichoke gives you a quarter of your daily fiber needs. In addition, it is extremely high in vitamin C, potassium, folic acid, magnesium, and other minerals. And unless you dip it in butter, the artichoke is fat-free and low in calories.

There's another good reason to become an artichoke lover — to lower your cholesterol. In one study, people with high cholesterol received artichoke juice instead of cholesterol-lowering drugs. Their LDL (bad) cholesterol, total cholesterol, and triglyceride levels fell an average of 8 percent, while their HDL (good) cholesterol levels increased. Those on traditional medicines lowered their cholesterol levels only a few percentage points more.

Other researchers have noticed that artichokes improve blood fat levels overall. It seems that something in the artichoke stimulates the liver into producing more bile. The bile grabs fat molecules, allowing the enzymes in the intestines to digest them. More bile means less fat in your bloodstream.

The next time you're at the grocery store toss an artichoke in your cart and make your heart happy.

Aspirin

Powerful heart protection in one little pill

Aspirin may be the safest, cheapest, most effective way to fight heart attack and stroke. And even though today, this little pill is almost more famous for its heart benefits than as a headache remedy, it hasn't always enjoyed such widespread praise.

Since the time of Hippocrates, willow bark was used for a variety of aches and pains. Its key ingredient, salicylic acid, was eventually isolated and produced, but it caused such stomach irritation that many people found the cure worse than the condition. It wasn't until the late 1800s that Bayer, a small company in Germany, synthesized acetylsalicylic acid and came up with what we call aspirin. Today, it's a staple in almost every medicine cabinet. Over 80 billion aspirin are taken by Americans each year. It's also the main ingredient in more than 50 over-the-counter products.

Within the last decade, aspirin therapy has become a commonly prescribed treatment for those who have suffered a heart attack or are at risk of one. Salicylic acid, the active part of aspirin, keeps blood cells from clumping to each other and sticking to the walls of your arteries. This reduces the risk of blood clots and heart attacks.

Aspirin therapy involves taking small doses, one 81-milligram (mg) baby aspirin, every day to help your blood remain clot-free. However, the latest research now says a booster dose twice a month might be necessary for this type of therapy to stay effective. It seems that a larger dose, about 325 mg or one regular aspirin, keeps the blood cells from telling platelets to form clots. After about two weeks, that dose wears off and another one is needed. Experts recommend a 325-mg dose on the 1st and 15th of each month and a smaller, 81-mg dose the rest of the month.

Talk to your doctor about aspirin therapy if you are a man over 40 or a woman over 50 and have one of the following heart disease risk factors:

- smoking
- family history of early heart attack
- high blood pressure
- high cholesterol
- diabetes
- postmenopausal but not on hormone replacement therapy

Increase your odds of surviving a heart attack

Although many doctors recommend long-term aspirin use for those at risk of heart disease, more people need to know about its immediate, life-saving benefits in the case of a heart attack. Dr. Charles Hennekens, professor of medicine at Harvard Medical School in Boston, recommends taking a 325 mg aspirin at the first sign of a heart attack — chest pain that spreads into your jaw, arm, or back. According to the American Heart Association, 5,000 to 10,000 lives could be saved every year if this immediate treatment were more widely practiced. But remember, call 911 first and then take an aspirin.

A word of warning for travelers — since not all airliners have aspirin on board, be sure and pack some in your carry-on luggage. Chest pain at 30,000 feet is nothing to take lightly, so be prepared.

🐌 🐌 🐌

When you shouldn't take aspirin

Aspirin can make certain health conditions worse. Check with your doctor before taking aspirin if you have:
- gout
- stomach ulcers
- liver disease
- history of hemorrhagic stroke
- history of cerebral aneurysm
- uncontrolled high blood pressure
- asthma
- nasal polyps

🐌 🐌

Heart attack and infection: What's the connection?

New research has uncovered some startling possibilities about aspirin and its role in heart disease.

In the well-known Physicians' Health Study, scientists measured the relationship between inflammation inside the arteries, the incidence of heart attacks, and the effects of aspirin.

They found that a chronic type of inflammation, possibly caused by a viral infection, goes hand-in-hand with a heart attack. People with the most inflammation were three times more likely to have a heart attack and twice as likely to suffer a stroke. Because the inflamed arteries are so narrowed, they could restrict blood flow enough to trigger a heart attack.

Aspirin therapy reduced heart attacks in the highest risk group by more than 55 percent. This suggests another important benefit from aspirin — fighting inflammation in your arteries.

See the *Germ warfare* chapter for more information on bad "bugs" that can hurt your heart.

Get the benefits of aspirin from the food you eat

You would never consider crumbling an aspirin on top of your ice cream or onto your toothbrush. What about swirling one into your pudding or dissolving one in your soda? Sound unappetizing? Don't worry ... no one is recommending you do any of these things. You can, however, get the same heart benefits of aspirin from the foods you eat.

It started back in the 1950s, when shipping and food storage methods began to improve. As a result, perishable fruits such as oranges, cherries, and berries became more widely available year-round throughout the United States. About the same time, doctors began to see fewer deaths from heart disease.

But it wasn't until the last decade that scientists put these two events together and came up with a heart-healthy link. The same substance, salicylic acid, that is the active part of acetyl-salicylic acid or aspirin, also occurs naturally in many foods.

Aspirin is quite good at controlling blood clots by keeping platelets from clumping for their entire life span, about 10 days. The salicylates in foods are not as powerful and their effects are more temporary. But it's easy to take in a small, steady supply of salicylates through the foods you eat.

Although fresh foods are the best choice because they contain all kinds of important nutrients, you can get salicylates from other foods, too. Manufacturers have been using them for flavoring, aroma, and as preservatives in hundreds of processed foods for about 30 years. These are called synthetic salicylates, and they can be beneficial for your heart, as well.

Foods with natural salicylates	Apricots, Cantaloupes, Dates, Grapes, Oranges, Pineapple, Raisins, Raspberries
Dried herbs high in salicylates	Thyme, Paprika, Garam masala, Cumin, Dill, Oregano, Turmeric, Curry powder
Processed foods with synthetic salicylates	Ice cream, Gelatin, Pudding, Chewing gum, Syrup, Candy, Beverages, Baked goods
Common flavorings with synthetic salicylates	Fruit (peach, grape, etc.), Mint, Wintergreen, Caramel, Butter, Cinnamon, Nut, Root beer, Vanilla

Researchers think you could be eating anywhere from 10 to 220 mg of salicylates every day, from those occurring naturally in some foods and the synthetic type added to processed foods and flavorings.

A word of caution

Some people are particularly sensitive to salicylates and can have reactions ranging from nausea and dizziness to hives, internal bleeding, and hyperventilation. If you know you are aspirin-sensitive, talk to your doctor before beginning aspirin therapy. You may even need to go through an "elimination diet," a program that gradually eliminates foods containing salicylates.

🐜 🐜 🐜

Aspirin helps defuse an 'angry' heart

If you've ever gotten so mad you felt like you were just going to explode, don't underestimate the risk. Your arteries could, in fact, have a mini-explosion, leading to vessel damage, clotting, and perhaps even a heart attack.

A Harvard Medical School study of over a thousand men and women revealed that episodes of anger can double your risk of a heart attack, even up to two hours after the angry outburst. Researchers also discovered that the people in this study who were regular aspirin users had a significantly lower risk of heart attack.

So, while you still need to learn how to deal with your anger, it's nice to know a little aspirin can at least reduce anger's deadly side effect.

See the *Anger arresters* chapter for natural ways to take charge of your emotions.

Avocados

6 heart-smart reasons to eat an avocado

Gives bad fats the brush-off. Your body needs some fat — but only the good kind, like monounsaturated and some polyunsaturated fats. About two-thirds of the fat in an avocado is monounsaturated fat, the same heart-healthy kind found in olive oil. Avocados are also a good source of vitamin E.

Just remember, avocados contain some saturated fat. Eat them in moderation and in place of other high-fat foods, such as butter, cheese, and sour cream.

Helps conquer bad cholesterol. Several studies have shown that avocados can improve cholesterol levels. When avocados were eaten as a main source of monounsaturated fat in an otherwise low-fat diet, bad LDL cholesterol levels went down and good HDL cholesterol went up. In fact, adding avocados to your weekly menu may be better for your cholesterol than loading up on complex carbohydrates, like starches and fiber.

The secret may lie in the large amounts of linoleic and linolenic acids in avocados. You can only get these two polyunsaturated fatty acids from your diet, yet they are necessary for important heart functions, like controlling blood pressure, blood clotting, and blood fat levels. One avocado provides more than half your daily requirement of linoleic acid.

Increases folic acid. Avocados are a particularly good source of folic acid. This B vitamin neutralizes the bad effects of homocysteine, a byproduct of protein metabolism that damages and narrows your arteries. Folic acid is found in many plant foods, although much of it is destroyed during cooking or processing. Since avocados are usually eaten raw, they provide a healthy dose of folic acid, as well as the other B vitamins.

Beefs up antioxidants. This tasty fruit is high in lots of vitamins, especially C and E, two important weapons against free radicals. By working as antioxidants, vitamins C and E keep free radicals from reacting with the cholesterol in your blood. As a result, the cholesterol is less likely to attach to the walls of your arteries and form plaques.

Boosts fiber intake. If you want to eat more fiber, avocados provide a delicious alternative. One medium avocado has more fiber than almost any other fruit, almost 5 grams. That's about as much fiber as you'll get in a cup of raisin bran cereal. Fiber helps your body get rid of cholesterol before it has a chance to do any damage.

Maximizes your minerals. If you're looking for a great source of minerals, look no further than this wrinkled fruit. Each one is a great source of iron, magnesium, manganese, and copper. And don't forget potassium, a mineral that is extremely important to good heart health. One avocado contains twice as much potassium as a banana.

B vitamins

Battle heart disease with B vitamins

Your heart has a new enemy. You've known for years that high levels of cholesterol were bad for your heart. Now research finds that an amino acid called homocysteine pairs up with cholesterol to make having a healthy heart even tougher.

Luckily, researchers have discovered weapons you can use to fight homocysteine. And these weapons can be found in the food you eat every day. A trio of B vitamins — folic acid, vitamin B6, and vitamin B12 — team up to convert homocysteine into a less-dangerous substance.

Folic acid is so important in neutralizing the bad effects of homocysteine that experts estimate about 40 percent of heart attacks and strokes suffered by men in the United States may be caused by a folic acid deficiency.

Women aren't exempt from the dangers of homocysteine either. A recent study found that women who got the most folic acid and vitamin B6, either from supplements or from their diets, were much less likely to develop heart disease.

Homocysteine isn't harmful to you in normal amounts. It's made from another amino acid, methionine, during the process of metabolizing protein. Afterward, it should be turned back into methionine, but here's the catch — it needs B vitamins, especially folic acid, to be converted back to its original form. If you don't have enough B vitamins to do the job, homocysteine can build up to dangerous levels, which can damage your arteries and lead to heart disease and stroke.

Because homocysteine is a by-product of protein metabolism, people who eat high-protein diets should take special care to get plenty of B vitamins.

Recommended dietary allowance (RDA)

	Folic acid	B12	B6
Males ages 19-50	400 mcg	2.4 mcg	1.3 mg
Males ages 51-up	400 mcg	2.4 mcg	1.7 mg
Females ages 19-50	400 mcg	2.4 mcg	1.3 mg
Females ages 51-up	400 mcg	2.4 mcg	1.5 mg
Pregnant	600 mcg	2.6 mcg	1.9 mg

Balancing your Bs the key to good health

There are many B vitamins — thiamin (B1), riboflavin (B2), niacin (B3), pantothenic acid (B5), pyridoxine (B6), cobalamin (B12), folic acid, and biotin — and they often work together. It is very unusual to have a deficiency of just one B vitamin. For example, your body requires folic acid in order to absorb the other B vitamins. A deficiency of folic acid could quickly lead to deficiencies in the other B vitamins as well.

To be sure you're getting all of the B vitamins, vary your diet to include meats or other sources of protein with plenty of fresh fruits and vegetables. Keep in mind that folic acid, vitamin B6, and vitamin B12 are especially important for heart and artery health.

Folic acid. This vitamin took its name from the word foliage, so as you might expect, it's found mostly in plant foods. Legumes, like pinto beans, and leafy green vegetables, like spinach, are particularly good sources. Cooking and processing can reduce the amount of folic acid in your food, so stick to fresh and raw foods whenever possible.

Drugs can sometimes interfere with your body's ability to absorb folic acid. The most common offenders include aspirin, antacids, oral contraceptives, and anticonvulsants. Other things that can deplete your body's supply of folic acid include alcoholism, tobacco use, stress, pregnancy, and breastfeeding.

Vitamin B6. If you eat beans to get folic acid and meat to get vitamin B12, make sure you also get plenty of vitamin B6. Those foods are high in protein, and B6 is particularly important to your body in processing protein properly.

Vitamin B12. This energy-supplying vitamin can only be found in foods of animal origin, like meat and dairy products, so vegetarians have a higher risk of becoming deficient.

Food	Folic acid	Vitamin B12	Vitamin B6
Spinach, 1 cup	262 mcg	0	.45 mg
Pinto beans, 1 cup	294 mcg	0	.27 mg
Beef liver, fried, 3 ounces	187 mcg	95 mcg	1.2 mg
Avocado, 1 Florida	162 mcg	0	.85 mg
Salmon, smoked, 3 ounces	1.62 mcg	2.77 mcg	.24 mg
Sirloin steak, broiled, 3 ounces	7.65 mcg	2.23 mcg	.33 mg
Milk, whole, 1 cup	12.2 mcg	.87 mcg	.10 mg
Ground beef, fried, 3 ounces	7.65 mcg	2.30 mcg	.20 mg
Lima beans, 1 cup	44.7 mcg	0	.33 mg

Food *(continued)*	Folic acid	Vitamin B12	Vitamin B6
Yogurt, plain, 8 ounces	16.8 mcg	.84 mcg	.07 mg
Potato, baked, 1 medium	14.2 mcg	0	.47 mg
Asparagus, 1/2 cup	131 mcg	0	.11 mg
Green peas, 1 cup	101 mcg	0	.35 mg
Banana, 1	21.8 mcg	0	.66 mg

Heal stroke damage with B vitamins

Studies have shown that B vitamins can help lower your risk of suffering a heart attack or stroke. Now a new study has found that taking B vitamins after a stroke may also help heal the damage.

Researchers divided 50 stroke survivors into two groups. One group took a vitamin supplement containing 1 mg of vitamin B12, 100 mg of vitamin B6, and 5 mg of folic acid. The other group took a vitamin supplement without the B vitamins.

After three months, the people who were taking the vitamin supplements with the B vitamins had lower levels of homocysteine and thrombomodulin, a chemical indicator of blood vessel damage.

Researchers don't know if the results mean that B vitamins may help prevent a second stroke, but more studies are planned to uncover the complete role B vitamins play in your health.

Beware — some vitamins can be toxic

The B vitamins are water-soluble, so most of them are considered safe, even in large doses. That's because any excess usually just passes out of your body in your urine.

However, B6 is an exception to the rule. It can be toxic in doses of 200 mg or more, causing bone pain and muscle weakness. Very large doses may cause permanent nerve damage.

Asparagus Salad and Pecans

24 medium-sized fresh asparagus spears
6 crisp lettuce leaves
6 tablespoons nonfat ranch salad dressing
2 tablespoons chopped pecans, lightly toasted

Bring a large pot of water to boil. Wash asparagus; snap off tough bottoms of stems. Add asparagus and let water return to a boil. Cook about 3 minutes, until asparagus is crisp but tender. Remove asparagus, run under cold water or immerse in ice water, then refrigerate until chilled.

At serving time, line six salad plates with lettuce, and arrange 4 asparagus spears on each. Top each salad with 1 tablespoon dressing, and sprinkle with 1 teaspoon toasted pecans.

Makes 6 servings

Per serving: 32 Calories; 1g Fat (0g from saturated fat) (26% calories from fat); 1g Protein; 5g Carbohydrate; 0mg Cholesterol; 151mg Sodium

Reprinted with permission from The Art of Cooking for the Diabetic by Mary Abbott Hess, 1996

Bowtie Chicken Salad

1 1/2 cups cooked bowtie pasta
2 medium tomatoes, diced
8 ounces fresh asparagus, steamed and cut into 3-inch lengths
8 ounces boneless, skinless chicken breast, baked and cubed
4 green onions
1 cup diced green bell pepper
4 tablespoons nonfat Italian salad dressing
2 tablespoons balsamic vinegar
4 tablespoons grated Parmesan cheese

Toss all ingredients together in large mixing bowl. You can serve it right away or chill for later. Sprinkle the top with fresh cracked black pepper.

Variations:

Any small, shaped pasta (e.g. rotini, penne, or rotelle) may be substituted for the bowtie pasta.

Tuna canned in water can be substituted for the chicken.

Balsamic vinegar is an Italian aged vinegar which is dark in color and has a rich, mellow flavor. You can also substitute red wine vinegar.

Makes 4 servings

Per serving: 319 Calories; 4g Fat (1g from saturated fat) (10% calories from fat); 25g Protein; 52g Carbohydrate; 37mg Cholesterol; 374mg Sodium

This is an official 5 A Day Recipe. This recipe is provided by the National Institutes of Health. To serve this colorful salad, line your plates with dark green lettuce.

Mango and Melon Salad with Strawberry Sauce

1 fresh mango, peeled and sliced into bite-sized pieces
(see instructions below)
1/2 cantaloupe, peeled and sliced into bite-sized pieces
1/2 honeydew, peeled and sliced into bite-sized pieces
1 1/2 cups fresh strawberries, or partially thawed frozen
strawberries
1 tablespoon lemon juice
1/4 cup confectioners sugar

Place mango and melon pieces in a large serving bowl.

In a blender, blend strawberries with lemon juice and sugar
until smooth. Drizzle sauce over fruit salad and serve.

How to slice a mango:

Slice each side of the mango vertically along the seed to give
two halves, and pull them apart.

Hold one mango half, peel side down, and score the fruit
down to the peel (but not through it) in a tic-tac-toe fashion.

Hold the scored portion with both hands and bend the peel
backwards so that the "diamond cut" cubes are exposed.

Cut cubes off the peel, and then remove any remaining fruit
clinging to the seed.

Makes 4 servings

Per serving: 107 Calories; less than 1g Fat (4% calories from fat);
1g Protein; 27g Carbohydrate; 0mg Cholesterol; 12mg Sodium

*This is an official 5 A Day Recipe. This recipe is provided by the National
Institutes of Health. Although it sounds too delicious to be good for you, this
salad provides two servings of fruit for each person.*

Stuffed Baked Potato

4 baking potatoes, about 1/2 lb. each
1/2 cup low-fat cottage cheese
3 tablespoons skim milk
1 teaspoon chives, dried or fresh
1/8 teaspoon pepper
paprika, as desired

Preheat oven to 425 degrees F.

Wash and dry potatoes. Prick skins with fork. Bake potatoes until tender, 50 to 60 minutes. (Potatoes may be baked in a microwave oven. Use the directions that came with your oven.)

Beat cottage cheese until smooth.

Slice tops off potatoes. Scoop out insides of potatoes and add to cottage cheese. Add milk and seasonings. Beat until well-blended.

Stuff potato skins with potato-cheese mixture. Sprinkle with paprika.

Return potatoes to oven. Bake about 10 minutes or until heated and tops are lightly browned.

Makes 4 servings

Per serving: 114 Calories; less than one gram Fat (3% calories from fat); 6g Protein; 22g Carbohydrate; 1mg Cholesterol; 127mg Sodium

Butter vs. Margarine

Saturated or unsaturated?
Choose wisely to protect your heart

Foods cooked in butter or lard may taste great, but these animal fats can do bad things to your arteries. The latest controversy surrounding butter, margarine, and heart health has caused more than a few people to toss out the plastic tubs and run happily back to their butter dishes.

While it's true that research has proven certain margarines do contribute to high cholesterol and heart disease, check out these facts:

- **Butter** is the solid fat that comes from churning cream or whole milk. It's high in cholesterol and saturated fat. You can tell it contains saturated fat because it's solid at room temperature. Butter just loves to clog up your arteries. As strange as it seems, eating cholesterol doesn't raise blood cholesterol as much as eating foods high in saturated fat.

♦ **Margarine** is made mostly from unsaturated vegetable oil and, therefore, has no cholesterol. Unsaturated fats have been shown to reduce blood cholesterol levels. Margarine is often fortified with vitamins A and D. It softens but does not become liquid at room temperature, which means it contains only some saturated fat.

	Butter (1 tablespoon)	**Hard Margarine** (1 tablespoon)	**Softspread Margarine** (1 tablespoon)
Total fat	11 grams	11 grams	9 grams
Saturated fat	7.1 grams	2.2 grams	1.8 grams
Monounsaturated fat	3.3 grams	5 grams	4.4 grams
Polyunsaturated fat	.4 gram	3.6 grams	1.9 grams
Cholesterol	31 mg	0 mg	0 mg
Calcium	3 mg	4 mg	3 mg
Sodium	117 mg	132 mg	139 mg
Vitamin A	107 RE	139 RE	139 RE

Melting the margarine mystery

Up until the early 1900s, animal fats and tropical oils, like coconut oil and palm oil, were your only choice for baking, frying, or spreading. That meant lots of saturated fat. Then a process called hydrogenation was developed that took liquid vegetable oils, like cottonseed oil, and turned them into products that were solid, less likely to spoil, and could be used in all manner of cooking. By the 1960s, animal fat was being used for only about a third of our cooking needs, while hydrogenated vegetable oil products were used in the majority of kitchens across the country. Suddenly, we were consuming less saturated fat. Nutritionists and health experts rejoiced.

Then came the bad news. When vegetable oils are hardened during hydrogenation, trans fatty acids are formed. These trans fatty acids turn out to have the same effect in the body as saturated fat. That means they raise blood cholesterol levels.

Many people heard this news and immediately switched from margarine back to butter before considering all the facts.

- Butter is high in saturated fat and cholesterol.

- Hard, stick margarines, which are mostly hydrogenated oils, contain a large amount of trans fatty acids, but soft or liquid margarines contain little, if any, trans fatty acids.

Several studies have revealed that replacing butter with soft tub margarine reduces the risk of heart disease by 10 percent. Yet, replacing butter with hard, stick margarine has no effect at all.

You will find that most margarines today are made from a mixture of partially hydrogenated vegetable oil and liquid vegetable oil. Remember, the more solid the product is the more trans fatty acids it contains per ounce.

Here's the latest American Heart Association recommendation:

- Choose a margarine with no more than 2 grams of saturated fat per tablespoon.

- Look for a margarine with liquid vegetable oil listed as the first ingredient.

- Buy soft margarines instead of stick.

In addition, lowering your intake of total fat by eating reduced fat, low fat, and fat free versions of your favorite foods will not only keep the trans fats down but will improve your diet and your health overall.

How the spreads measure up

Margarines, fats, and oils (1 tablespoon)	Calories	Total fat (grams)	Sat fat (grams)	Trans fat (grams)
Promise Ultra Fat Free, tub	5	0	0	0
Smart Beat Fat Free! Smarter than Butter!, tub	15	0	0	0
Smart Beat Smarter than Fat Free Super Light Margarine, tub	20	2	0	0
Promise Ultra 70% Less Fat, tub	30	4	0	0
Fleischmann's Lower Fat Margarine, tub	40	5	0	0
Spectrum Naturals Spread, tub	90	11	1	0
Canola oil	120	14	1	0
Weight Watchers Light Margarine, tub	50	4	1	1
I Can't Believe It's Not Butter! Light, stick	50	6	1	1
Shedd's Spread Country Crock, tub	70	7	1	1
Promise, tub	90	10	2	0
Olive oil	120	14	2	0
Soybean oil	120	14	2	0
Land O' Lakes Light Whipped Butter	40	4	3	0
Land O' Lakes Country Morning Blend Light, stick or tub	50	6	3	0
Land O' Lakes Spread with Sweet Cream, tub	80	8	2	1
I Can't Believe It's Not Butter!, tub	90	10	2	1

Margarines, fats, and oils (1 tablespoon)	Calories	Total fat (grams)	Sat fat (grams)	Trans fat (grams)
Promise, stick	90	10	2	2
Land O' Lakes Country Morning Blend Margarine, tub	100	11	2	1
Land O' Lakes Spread with Sweet Cream, stick	90	10	2	2
Parkay, stick	90	10	2	3
Land O' Lakes Country Morning Blend Margarine, stick	100	11	2	2
Land O' Lakes Margarine, stick or tub	100	11	2	2
Crisco, can	110	12	3	1
Chicken fat	120	13	4	0
Land O' Lakes Sweet Cream Whipped Butter	60	7	5	0
Lard	120	13	5	0
Butter	100	11	7	0
Beef tallow	120	13	6	0

Easy way to uncover hidden trans fats

Before you put a box of crackers or a package of donuts in your shopping cart, read the label. Even though the Food and Drug Administration (FDA) does not require manufacturers to list trans fats separately on food labels, you can still get a clue from the other ingredients.

If you see hydrogenated vegetable oil on the ingredient list, there's a good chance the product contains trans fats. Even partially hydrogenated oils contain small amounts of trans fatty acids.

Why do manufacturers continue to use hydrogenated oils? They say their products stay fresher and have a better texture and quality with these oils.

But public outcry against trans fats could force food manufacturers to list how much of these fats are in their products. This could also encourage them to decrease the amount of trans fats they use and to find healthier alternatives.

❧ ❧ ❧

Clobber cholesterol with new margarine

A margarine you can spread on your toast that reduces cholesterol? It may sound too good to be true, but this is not science fiction.

The first new margarine substitute contains sitostanol ester, a by-product of the wood processing industry, which has been proven to lower cholesterol. A company in Finland was the first to introduce this ground-breaking margarine, but McNeil Consumer Products Co., a subsidiary of Johnson & Johnson, has licensed sitostanol ester in the United States. Their product, Benecol, contains sitostanol in a canola oil-based margarine.

Another heart-healthy spread you may find in your local grocery is made from plant sterols extracted from soybeans. This one, called Take Control, is a Lipton foods product.

Both plant extracts lower LDL (bad) cholesterol by blocking how much cholesterol is absorbed into the bloodstream, which could reduce your need for cholesterol-lowering drugs. One study showed a 20 percent drop in LDL. Try that on your pancakes.   *❧ ❧*

Calcium and Dairy

3 great reasons to get more calcium

When you think of a healthy heart, do you think of calcium? Probably not, but many doctors all over the world think you should. They say it's not just for healthy teeth and bones anymore.

Beats high blood pressure. Although the benefit is small and calcium alone can't prevent or treat high blood pressure, drinking milk goes hand-in-hand with lower blood pressure. The reverse is true, as well. People with high blood pressure have low levels of calcium.

Researchers at the University of Southern California School of Medicine reported a 12 percent drop in high blood pressure risk for every gram of calcium consumed.

The exact relationship is still unclear, but researchers think there may be an unidentified heart-protective ingredient in calcium and certain other minerals, like potassium and magnesium. These minerals can help keep your blood pressure in balance even if your diet is too high in salt. Another theory is that calcium relaxes your arteries and allows more blood to flow through.

All you really need to know is this — if you want to reduce your risk of high blood pressure, get more calcium every day.

Cuts your risk of high cholesterol. Calcium plays an important role in controlling cholesterol. It teams up with saturated and other fats in your intestines and keeps your body from absorbing them. Fewer fats in your bloodstream mean lower cholesterol.

Gives your heart rhythm. As far as overall heart health is concerned, too little calcium, a condition called hypocalcemia, can cause serious problems. Since calcium helps control your heartbeat, not enough of this mineral in your body can cause an irregular heartbeat and possibly cardiac arrest. You are especially at risk if you have a severe burn or infection, inflammation of the pancreas, kidney failure, or damaged parathyroid glands.

Drinking milk can be a stroke of luck

Many times high blood pressure goes hand-in-hand with stroke. Since calcium helps control blood pressure, experts wondered if it would also reduce the risk of stroke.

Researchers looked at information on several thousand men compiled over 22 years. The risk of stroke was quite different between the men who took calcium pills and those who ate a lot of dairy products. Men who drank more than 16 ounces of milk a day were half as likely to suffer a stroke as those who didn't drink milk. Those who got their calcium from nondairy sources, such as supplements, had no stroke advantage.

Is it the natural calcium or is it the milk? What exactly gave these men that extra shot of protection? Puzzled scientists think these findings could mean there is an unidentified ingredient in milk that helps prevent stroke. It's also possible that drinking milk was simply one part of an overall healthier lifestyle of the test group.

Research shows most Americans don't get nearly enough calcium. The average daily intake is 500 to 700 mg a day, while the new recommended amount for postmenopausal women and men over 50 is 1,200 to 1,500 mg a day. That means most people need to double the amount of calcium they take in. Remember, it's more than just your bones that are at stake. Strong and healthy arteries need calcium, too.

New milk labels mean better information for you

The last time you were reaching for your favorite gallon of milk, did you notice something different on your old carton? The Food and Drug Administration (FDA) has come out with some new labeling requirements that should make it easier for you to find and buy the milk you really want.

Old name	Possible new names	Total fat (grams)	% Daily Value*
Milk	Milk	8.0	12%
Low-fat 2 percent milk	Reduced-fat or less-fat milk	4.7	7%
(New product)	Light milk	4 or less	6% or less
Low-fat 1 percent milk	Low-fat milk	2.6	4%
Skim milk	Fat-free, skim, zero-fat, no-fat, or nonfat milk	less than 0.5	0%

*The Daily Value for fat is 65 grams. This means you should not eat more than 65 grams of fat each day — based on a 2,000 calorie diet.

Many people in the milk industry are happy about the changes for several reasons. They think some people don't drink skim milk because the name "skim" sounds less nutritious, even though only the fat has been removed, not the calcium or other important nutrients. Skim milk is, in fact, the number one choice of many health experts.

Also, these new labels allow manufacturers room to introduce new products, such as flavored milks and protein-enriched formulas.

Nutritionists hope more people will now choose products that are lower in saturated fat.

No matter what the carton looks like, drink three 8-ounce glasses of milk a day to help meet the recommended daily allowance of calcium.

🐦 🐦

Deciding the dairy defense that's right for you

	Amount	Calcium (mg)	Saturated fat (gm)	Cholesterol (mg)	Calories
Cheddar cheese, shredded	1 cup	815	24	119	455
Plain low-fat yogurt	8 oz	415	2	14	144
1% low-fat milk	1 cup	352	3	19	137
Fruit low-fat yogurt	8 oz	345	2	10	231
Skim milk	1 cup	302	.3	4	86
2% low-fat milk	1 cup	297	3	18	121
Whole milk	1 cup	291	5	33	150
Plain whole milk yogurt	8 oz	274	5	29	139
Cream cheese	3 oz	68	19	93	297

Make sure you look at all the columns in this chart before heading to the store. Cheddar cheese is rich in calcium, but it's also highest in saturated fat and cholesterol. And as you can see, whole milk contains the most saturated fat out of all the milks. That means it raises your cholesterol and clogs your arteries. Choose the lower fat varieties instead.

If you're looking to increase your calcium, don't depend on cream cheese. It contains little calcium compared to other dairy products, and it's fairly high in saturated fat. Butter and cream are also poor nutritional choices. They are almost pure fat and contain very little calcium.

A dairy alternative your heart will love

Maybe you love milk, but milk doesn't love you. If you are lactose intolerant, you are missing an important enzyme that helps your body digest milk and other dairy products. The result can be uncomfortable cramping and bloating. Thanks to new technology, you can now buy milk-like beverages that look and taste very similar to cow's milk but are made from grains.

Soy milk has been around for some time (see the *Soy* chapter for more information), but now oat and other grain products are becoming more popular.

Oat drinks are usually made from an oat base, with water, oil, vitamins, and flavoring added. They are 100 percent nondairy, contain no lactose, and are low in sodium. And there's more good news. Since they are a plant product, you don't have to worry about saturated animal fat and cholesterol. Your heart will love these grain beverages because adding oat products to your daily menu is a proven way to lower cholesterol. In fact, one study showed a 17 percent drop in bad LDL cholesterol when oat bran was added to a low-fat diet.

So pour them on cereal, stir them into coffee, or use them in cooking and baking. You'll be getting a heart-healthy dose of fiber while lowering your cholesterol.

To find these healthy dairy alternatives, visit your local
health food store or the health section of your favorite grocer.
Some brand names you may find are Mill Milk, West Brae,
Pacific, and Harmony Farms.

🐜 🐜 🐜

6 easy ways to eat less fat and get more calcium

- Low-fat cottage cheese may be low in fat, but it's also
  low in calcium (1/2 cup contains only 70 mg) and high
  in sodium (460 mg), making it a poor choice for a
  healthy heart and strong bones. Try some part skim
  ricotta instead — 1/2 cup has 334 mg of calcium.

- Add your own fruit to low-fat plain yogurt for the lowest
  fat, calories, and sugar. Fruited, whole milk yogurt has
  the least amount of calcium and the highest amount of
  calories of all the yogurts.

- When a recipe calls for mayonnaise or sour cream, sub
  stitute the same amount of nonfat plain yogurt.

- Most processed cheese and cheese spreads are high in
  sodium and low in calcium. If you must buy these, at
  least get the low-fat version.

- Natural cheese from part skim milk is low in fat and
  gives you a good dose of calcium. You can reduce the fat
  content of your favorite cheese simply by zapping it in
  the microwave for a minute or two, then pouring off any
  oil you can.

- Choose sherbets and frozen yogurt instead of ice cream
  if you want to watch your fat intake, but realize they are
  still full of sugar and calories. For the most calcium-rich
  frozen dessert, scoop out some frozen yogurt.

🐜 🐜

Cook up a broth loaded with calcium

If you can't or won't drink milk, don't despair. There's another rich source of calcium that's right in your own kitchen. It's not a dairy product — it's all those bones you normally throw into the trash.

Many Eastern cultures don't drink milk at all, yet they still get plenty of calcium throughout their lives. They do it by making stock out of chicken, turkey, fish, or pork bones. Here's how:

- Crack the bones.

- Soak them in vinegar.

- Boil them slowly until the bones become soft.

- Strain and use the liquid instead of water or commercial stock in stews, soups, and to cook vegetables or rice.

The acid in the vinegar draws out the calcium in the bones, yet most of the strong taste of the vinegar boils off. You are left with a stock so mineral-rich that one tablespoon contains over 100 milligrams (mg) of calcium.

Feast on calcium-rich fruits and vegetables

Experts believe ancient man got two or three times the amount of calcium from his diet than modern man. That's because he ate more plant foods. Today, only 6 percent of our total calcium comes from fruits and vegetables.

Some vegetables are high in calcium, but don't actually provide any to your body. That's because a certain chemical in foods like spinach, rhubarb, and Swiss chard keep the calcium from being absorbed. That doesn't mean you shouldn't eat these healthy vegetables — they still provide lots of nutrients. Just don't rely on them for your daily dose of calcium.

These fresh and processed fruits and vegetables are rich in calcium:

legumes	parsley
collards	kale
broccoli	tofu
dried figs	almonds

Calcium supplement lowers cholesterol

You know calcium supplements fight osteoporosis, but did you know that little pill can lower your cholesterol, as well. In a small study, researchers discovered that 1,200 mg of calcium carbonate a day, in addition to a low-fat, low-cholesterol diet, reduced bad LDL cholesterol by more than 4 percent and raised good HDL cholesterol by 4 percent.

If you decide to take supplements, be aware that manufacturers list the total weight of each pill, not the amount of pure calcium each contains. For instance, if you take a 600 mg tablet of calcium carbonate, you are getting only 240 mg of elemental or pure calcium. A 600 mg tablet of calcium citrate has only 144 mg of calcium.

Don't take more than 500 mg of pure calcium at once — your body can't absorb any more than that. You might have to do some math to figure this one out, but it's important.

Here are the most common types of calcium. Pick the one that is right for you.

calcium carbonate	40% calcium	economical, difficult to absorb so must be taken with food
calcium citrate	24% calcium	more expensive, easier to absorb
calcium gluconate	9% calcium	most expensive, difficult to break down

A lot of advertising phrases don't mean a thing. Ignore labels that say "no preservatives," "yeast-free," "all natural," "no starch," "no sugar," or "high potency," since these terms apply to all calcium supplements. But make sure you see "USP" on the label. This means the supplement meets U.S. Pharmacopoeia's dissolving and dosage standards.

Avoid high-fiber breads and cereals and aluminum-containing antacids when taking your calcium supplement. These keep your body from absorbing the mineral properly. In addition, certain medications, such as tetracycline, iron supplements, and thyroid hormones, can interfere with calcium absorption. Talk to your doctor.

Make sure your calcium supplement doesn't contain lead, especially if you are using natural sources, such as bone meal, dolomite, or oyster shell.

Although it's rare, you can have side effects from taking calcium supplements at normal dosages. Check with your doctor if you experience drowsiness, upset stomach, or difficult urination.

People who take too much calcium, several grams a day, risk serious problems, including kidney stones, severe constipation, and weakness. Extremely large overdoses can disrupt the acid/alkaline balance of your body and result in heartbeat irregularities and confusion.

Important calcium partners

Zinc. Your body is a complex machine where every nutrient you take in interacts with something else. Calcium is no different. If you take a calcium supplement with a meal, you could be decreasing your body's ability to absorb zinc by as much as 50 percent. It may be wise to eat more zinc if you plan on taking a calcium supplement. You can get lots of zinc by eating black beans, crab meat, steak, and oysters.

Magnesium. Like so many minerals, magnesium plays an important role in your body's delicate balance. If you don't have enough magnesium, your bones don't absorb calcium as efficiently. In fact, the calcium can end up deposited in the soft tissues of your body instead of your bones. Tests have shown that if you take in the proper amount of magnesium, calcium levels in your body rise, even if you don't take calcium supplements. For more magnesium, eat tofu, raisins, beans, peas, grains, green leafy vegetables, avocados, and nuts and seeds. If you plan on taking a supplement, buy the buffered form, like magnesium gluconate or citrate, to protect your digestive system. To make life simpler, you can even buy calcium/magnesium combinations.

Vitamin D. Watch your vitamin D, too, since it plays an important role in how much calcium your bones actually absorb. Eat eggs and shrimp, and drink fortified milk to get your calcium at the same time. When your body is exposed to sunshine, it makes its own vitamin D. But remember, during the winter or when using sunscreen, you are exposed to less sunshine, which means less vitamin D.

Chinese Peach Blossoms

2 pitted peaches, peeled and cubed
1 teaspoon lemon juice
1 cup plain yogurt
2 tablespoons frozen orange juice concentrate
brewer's yeast, optional

Prepare the peaches, covering them with the lemon juice until ready.

Put the peaches, yogurt, and orange juice concentrate in a blender and whirl 30 seconds at medium speed. If you want to have this concoction for an "instant breakfast," you might add some brewer's yeast.

Makes 2 servings

Per serving: 127 Calories; 4g Fat (2g from saturated fat) (26% calories from fat); 5g Protein; 20g Carbohydrate; 14mg Cholesterol; 53mg Sodium

Reprinted with permission from
Yogurt, Yoghurt, Youghourt: An International Cookbook
Food Products Press, An Imprint of The Haworth Press, Inc., 1995

Hearty Health Drink

2 tablespoons frozen orange juice concentrate
2 tablespoons blackstrap molasses
2 tablespoons safflower oil
1 teaspoon vanilla extract
1 cup plain yogurt
2 cups skim milk
1/2 cup dry milk
1/3 cup brewer's yeast

In an electric blender combine the juice concentrate, molasses, oil, vanilla, and yogurt. Blend at high speed for 1 minute. Add the milk, nonfat dry milk, and brewer's yeast and blend at medium speed for about 30 seconds more.

Makes 3 servings

Per serving: 317 Calories; 12g Fat (3g from saturated fat) (34% calories from fat); 18g Protein; 36g Carbohydrate; 15mg Cholesterol; 197mg Sodium

Reprinted with permission from
Yogurt, Yoghurt, Youghourt: An International Cookbook
Food Products Press, An Imprint of The Haworth Press, Inc., 1995

Arabic "Laban" Dressing

2 cloves garlic, minced
1 cup plain yogurt
1 teaspoon vegetable oil
1 teaspoon lemon juice or vinegar
salt and pepper to taste

Blend the garlic into the yogurt, then add the oil, lemon juice or vinegar, salt, and pepper. Serve on salad greens or as a topping for fried vegetables.

Makes 6 servings

Per serving: 31 Calories; 2g Fat (1g from saturated fat) (56% calories from fat); 1g Protein; 2g Carbohydrate; 5mg Cholesterol; 18mg Sodium

Reprinted with permission from
Yogurt, Yoghurt, Youghourt: An International Cookbook
Food Products Press, An Imprint of The Haworth Press, Inc., 1995

Canola Oil and Olive Oil

Natural clot-buster from your pantry

Just spoonfuls of canola oil offer big doses of protection from life-threatening blood clots. If you are at risk of a heart attack or stroke, canola oil, also known as rapeseed oil, can boost your body's defenses. Here's how it works.

Alpha-linolenic acid (ALA) is one of the polyunsaturated fats in canola oil. In fact, canola oil has more ALA than any other oil. This particular fatty acid discourages your blood from clumping together. If your blood doesn't clump, it won't form clots. Fewer clots mean a lower chance of suffering a heart attack or stroke.

But what about cholesterol? Canola can make a difference here, too. You've heard how a serving of salmon or herring is great for your heart — all those omega-3 fatty acids working hard to lower your bad cholesterol. But now you can get the same protection in less than 2 ounces of canola oil a day. That's great news if you're not a fish lover. Simply stir-fry that chicken in canola oil and watch your cholesterol drop.

6 reasons to cook with canola

- It's light-tasting with no distinctive flavor to overpower your foods.

- Canola won't separate from other salad dressing ingredients.

- It has the lowest amount of saturated fat of any oil.

- It's very high in monounsaturated fat, which helps balance your body's cholesterol.

- It contains omega-3 fatty acids, which lower cholesterol and triglycerides.

- It's cholesterol free.

On the horizon — a super canola plant

Here's one more example of how science hopes to improve upon Mother Nature.

Canola oil contains small amounts of stearic acid, a little less than 2 grams in every 100 grams of oil. This fatty acid has been studied by a number of nutrition experts. They say it reduces the amount of LDL cholesterol in your bloodstream and helps your liver produce less VLDL, the forerunner of bad cholesterol.

Now that scientists know stearic acid can be beneficial in controlling cholesterol, they want to make it easier for you to get more of it. By playing with the genetic makeup of the canola plant, they hope to come up with a strain that is higher in this cholesterol-clobbering element. Be on the lookout for this super canola plant sometime in the future.

A guide to heart-smart substitutions

If your recipe calls for a melted solid fat, such as butter or hard shortening, use this handy chart to substitute a healthier oil — like canola. Remember though, using canola instead of hard fats will make your food softer and more moist.

Melted solid fat	Canola oil
1 cup	3/4 cup
3/4 cup	2/3 cup
1/2 cup	1/3 cup
1/4 cup	3 tablespoons

Saturated or unsaturated: Which fat robs you of good health?

Saturated fats are the villains in today's cholesterol war. They raise your cholesterol and offer no heart-healthy benefits. Avoid high saturated fat foods whenever possible. These include meat, egg yolks, milk, butter, cheese, as well as a few vegetable fats like coconut oil, palm oil, and hydrogenated vegetable shortenings.

Polyunsaturated fats are the middle-of-the-road fats. They lower bad LDL cholesterol, which is good, but they also lower good HDL cholesterol, which is bad. A little of this kind of fat in your diet is all right, just don't overdo it. Safflower oil, sunflower oil, and soybean oil are high in polyunsaturates.

Monounsaturated fats are the good guys. These fats lower LDL cholesterol and can raise HDL cholesterol. Olive oil and canola oil are high in monounsaturated fats.

Olive oil — an ancient cure with up-to-date heart benefits

It's old news. The Greeks have known it for more than 6,000 years. It's been written about in the Bible. And now, finally, the Western world has taken these teachings to heart. Straight to their hearts.

Study after study has proven that olive oil lowers bad LDL cholesterol and raises good HDL cholesterol. This reduces your risk of heart disease. In fact, adding olive oil to a low-fat diet produces better results than just cutting out fat — thanks to the monounsaturated fat in olive oil.

If you look at the following chart, you'll see there are other oils high in monounsaturated fats. You might think these would be just as healthy as olive or canola oil, but that's not necessarily the case. In a small study, researchers in Spain tested sunflower oil against olive oil. Just as they had hoped, both raised HDL levels. But to their surprise, blood pressures in the olive oil group dropped as well.

Dietary fat source	Saturated fat %	Polyunsaturated fat %	Monounsaturated fat %
Canola oil	7	32	61
Safflower oil	10	76	14
Sunflower oil	12	72	16
Corn oil	13	58	29
Olive oil	15	10	75
Soybean oil	15	62	23
Peanut oil	19	33	48
Cottonseed oil	27	54	19
Lard	43	10	47
Beef tallow	48	3	49
Palm oil	51	10	39
Butterfat	68	4	28
Coconut oil	91	2	7

Earn kitchen honors with olive oil

Olive oil not only has the highest amount of monounsaturated fat of any oil, it's a good source of vitamin E. Cooks love olive oil because it won't break down into trans fatty acids at high heat, and it's cholesterol free. This fragrant oil has an intense flavor, which means you can use less. At 115 calories a tablespoon, that adds up to fewer calories. Another great benefit is its long shelf life. Stored in a dark, cool place, olive oil should keep its flavor for up to two years.

Solve the olive oil labeling mystery

You've seen them lining the store shelves, pretty bottles filled with golden, clear liquid, featuring exotic labels and confusing terms:

- extra virgin — a first-press oil considered to have the finest, most intense flavor; usually the most expensive; the flavor will break down at high temperatures so it's not recommended for frying

- fino or fine — a blend of extra virgin and virgin oils; good flavor but not as fruity

- light — contains the same amount of monounsaturated fat and calories as regular olive oil but has been filtered to lighten the color, fragrance, and flavor; good for baking and cooking without the distinctive olive oil taste; can be used for high-heat frying due to its higher smoke point

- pomace — oil extracted from the olive after the traditional pressing methods; heat and solvents are used to get this additional oil, which is then blended with virgin oil; less expensive than most varieties

- pure — an old term; now pure olive oil is simply labeled as olive oil and contains a combination of refined olive oil and virgin or extra virgin oil; use for frying and high-heat cooking

- refined — olive oil that must undergo a purifying process before it can be used; has no specific taste, odor, or color; combined with virgin oil to give it flavor

- virgin — a first-press oil not widely available in the United States

Basic Vinaigrette

1/3 cup red wine vinegar
1/2 teaspoon Dijon mustard
1/4 teaspoon salt
1/4 teaspoon freshly ground black pepper
1 cup olive oil

In a medium nonmetallic bowl, glass, or measuring cup, mix vinegar, mustard, salt, and pepper. Whisk olive oil in gradually to blend.
Variations:
Herb: Add 1/4 cup chopped parsley, dill, basil, oregano, or thyme, or a combination of herbs to the master recipe. Whisk to blend.
Garlic: Add 1 clove garlic, finely minced, to the master recipe.
Lemon juice: Substitute 1/4 cup fresh lemon juice plus 1 teaspoon grated lemon zest for red wine vinegar. Proceed with the master recipe.
Mustard: Add 2 teaspoons Dijon mustard.

Makes approximately 7 servings

Per serving: 275 Calories; 31g Fat (4g from saturated fat) (99% calories from fat); 0g Protein; 1g Carbohydrate; 0mg Cholesterol; 81mg Sodium

Reprinted courtesy of the International Olive Oil Council

Salmon Pasta Salad

1 can (15 1/2 ounces) Alaska salmon
8 ounces fusilli or macaroni, cooked, drained, and cooled
1 pint cherry tomatoes, halved
2 cups sliced cucumber
1 cup mozzarella cheese, cut into thin strips
1/2 cup chopped parsley
1/4 cup grated Parmesan cheese
Lemon Dressing

Drain and flake salmon. Toss flaked salmon with remaining ingredients in large serving bowl. Toss with Lemon Dressing and serve.

Lemon Dressing:

3/4 cup olive oil
1/4 cup lemon juice
2 cloves garlic, minced
1/2 teaspoon dill weed
1/2 teaspoon grated lemon peel
black pepper to taste

Whisk together ingredients until well combined.

Makes 8 servings

Per serving: 432 Calories; 28g Fat (6g from saturated fat) (59% calories from fat); 19g Protein; 25g Carbohydrate; 45mg Cholesterol; 418mg Sodium

Reprinted with permission from The Alaska Seafood Marketing Institute
www.state.ak.us/local/akpages/COMMERCE/asmihp.htm
Although higher in fat than some recipes, two-thirds of the fat is monounsaturated and rich in Omega-6

Veggie Pasta

2 red bell peppers
1 yellow bell pepper
12 medium mushrooms, sliced
6 ounces marinated artichoke hearts with liquid
1 medium onion, thinly sliced, separated into rings
24 cherry tomatoes, halved
2 teaspoons dried basil
4 cloves garlic, minced
1/2 teaspoon salt
6 tablespoons olive oil
2 tablespoons balsamic vinegar
15 olives, pitted and chopped
1/2 pound spaghetti

Broil peppers until skin is black and blistered on all sides. Remove and place in brown, paper bag for five minutes. When cool enough to handle, remove stem, seeds, and skin, and cut into strips. Place in a large bowl.

Add all other ingredients except spaghetti. Cover and marinate at room temperature for several hours or overnight in the refrigerator.

To assemble, cook spaghetti according to directions on the package. Heat veggies in microwave or gently in a large skillet over low heat, but do not cook them. Combine warm vegetables and pasta and serve immediately. Sprinkle with Parmesan cheese, if desired.

Makes 5 servings

Per serving: 547 Calories; 21g Fat (3g from saturated fat) (33% calories from fat); 16g Protein; 83g Carbohydrate; 0mg Cholesterol; 548mg Sodium

From The Vidalia Onion Cookbook

Cereal Grains

Great, golden grains — how to select a super heart-healthy cereal

Sitting down to a breakfast of bacon and eggs every morning has gone the way of crinolines and bobby socks. And probably just as well. Although that kind of breakfast may appeal to some, most people cringe at the thought of that much fat and cholesterol in one sitting.

Today, the breakfast of choice for many people is a bowl of cereal. And if you pour on low-fat milk, slice up a banana, and top it off with a glass of orange juice, so much the better. In fact, this is exactly the kind of breakfast health experts recommend.

But not all cereals are created equal. Many people like their cereal sweet, and manufacturers are more than happy to oblige. It is estimated that cereal makers use over 800 million pounds of sugar each year. If this surprises you, perhaps you haven't been reading those nutrition labels. Check out the numbers next time you reach for your favorite box. You'll have to weigh all the factors, though, since even some of the heavily sweetened cereals have extra B vitamins, iron, fiber, and calcium added in an effort to attract the health-conscious. And if getting enough folic acid is an issue, you'll be pleased to know that ready-to-eat cereals can be a major source.

The actual definition of cereal is any grain used for food, like wheat, oats, or rice. These make up more of your daily menu than you might think. If you were to combine all the different types of cereal grains eaten throughout the world, they would make up over half of the world's diet. But a more common meaning of cereal is any breakfast food made from grain. And if it's breakfast food you want, just take a trip down the cereal aisle of your local grocery store. You'll be amazed at the number and variety of boxed and bagged cereals, all proclaiming better taste, cuter shapes, or higher nutrition. The decision to buy can be agonizing. Here are some tips to help make it a bit easier.

- **Choose whole-grains.** You'll be fighting cholesterol and high blood pressure with every spoonful. Oats, buck wheat, whole wheat, and barley are super heart-healthy.

- **Read the labels.** Granolas, especially, are high in fat or saturated fatty acids.

- **Weigh the fruit.** It may be a trade-off. Many fruits such as apples, dates, and raisins are added to cereals for an extra taste punch. And while these fruits add some fiber, you have to decide if it's worth the extra sugar. For instance, one and a half ounces of raisins contain only 2 grams of fiber, but a whopping 30 grams of sugar. While it is a natural source of sugar, it's also in addition to whatever sugar coats your flakes. Your best bet is to choose an unsweetened cereal and add your own fruit.

- **Pass on the puffs.** If your cereal is mostly air, that's what your body will be getting.

- **Go for the slow.** Cooked oatmeal is a wonderfully warm way to start your morning. But in our hurried world, most people choose quick-cooking or instant oats, even though the slow-cooking variety has twice as much fiber. A very good reason to set your alarm a bit earlier.

Clobber cholesterol with cereal fiber

Whole grains contain all sorts of healthy things, like antioxidants, phytoestrogens, and starches, that nutritionists say can protect against cancer. But the biggest whole grain benefit is fiber. It not only fills you up so you eat less, it helps prevent constipation. Some experts think it might even help lower blood pressure. As if that wasn't enough, it blasts heart disease by lowering bad LDL cholesterol while keeping the levels of good HDL cholesterol steady.

Need proof? Over 40,000 men were involved in a six-year study exploring the relationship between fiber and heart disease. The researchers tested the three major sources of fiber — vegetables, fruits, and cereals — and found that cereal fiber had the biggest impact on heart health.

For every additional 10 grams of cereal fiber the men in the study ate each day, their risk of heart attack decreased dramatically — by almost 30 percent. That's a big benefit from a little fiber. To get about 10 grams of cereal fiber, you need to eat just one of the following:

1 cup oatmeal
1/2 cup All-Bran Extra Fiber
3 cups Cheerios
2 cups Complete Bran Flakes
1 cup Cracklin' Oat Bran
1 cup Grape Nuts
1 1/2 cups Kellogg's Low Fat Granola
4 biscuits Nabisco Shredded Wheat
3 cups Wheaties
3 packages Quaker Instant Oatmeal

The Food and Drug Administration (FDA) and the National Cancer Institute recommend you get about 25 grams of fiber every day. By starting your day with a hearty bowl of cereal, you'll be well on your way to reaching that goal. But don't stop there. Nutritionists say there is nothing wrong with grabbing cereal for an afternoon or evening snack. And if you need a quick meal after a hard day, cereal, milk or yogurt, and fruit is better for you than fast food or packaged snacks.

So let yourself go in the cereal aisle. Fill your cart with two or three or four boxes for variety — and crunch out cholesterol.

How to get more cereal fiber in your diet

- Sprinkle it on top of casseroles, soups, or baked potatoes
- Add some to muffin, biscuit, pancake, cake, or cookie mixes
- Top your yogurt or ice cream
- Blend up a better breakfast drink by mixing wheat germ into milk or juice
- Substitute crushed cereal for 1/4 to 1/3 of the crumb topping on a pie
- Toss some into fruit or green salads for extra crunch
- Use crushed cereal as a coating for baked fish or chicken
- Add to meatloaf or other ground meat dishes
- Combine chunky, high-fiber cereal with dried fruit and nuts for a tasty snack

Choose the right fiber for the right job

We live in the Information Age, a time when you are constantly bombarded with facts, theories, statistics, and opinions.

A time when having only a piece of information is as confusing as having too much.

Take fiber. You know it's good for you so you automatically grab whatever product label screams "high in fiber." But are you getting the right kind of fiber?

Plants are made up of two kinds of fiber — soluble and insoluble. Insoluble fiber doesn't dissolve in water. It speeds up your food's trip through your digestive system. That reduces your risk of colon cancer, diverticulosis, and appendicitis. It also keeps your stools soft and your bowels moving regularly. That helps prevent constipation, hemorrhoids, hiatal hernia, and irritable bowel syndrome. It also relieves some types of diarrhea. Since the fiber absorbs water and swells, you feel full long after you eat it. That helps you lose weight. Insoluble fiber is found in whole grains, wheat bran, vegetables, seeds, peas, beans, brown rice, and popcorn.

Soluble fiber dissolves easily in water. It can make food gummy or gel-like. It helps lower cholesterol and keeps blood sugar levels under control, even for people with diabetes. Fruits, vegetables, seeds, rye, oats, barley, rice bran, peas, and beans are good sources of soluble fiber.

Whole grain oats and barley are high in soluble and insoluble fiber.

Experts recommend you add both types of fiber to your diet, but do it gradually — over a three-week period. That way you'll avoid digestive problems like diarrhea, gas, and bloating. And don't forget to drink more water as you eat more fiber.

🐜 🐜 🐜

It's all in the label

The Daily Reference Value (DRV) for fiber is 25 grams, based on a 2,000 calorie diet. In order for a product to claim that it's a "good source" of fiber, it must contain at least 10 percent of the DRV, or 2.5 grams. If it contains at least 5 grams of fiber, or 20 percent of the DRV, the label may read "high" source.

High-fiber grains your heart will love

If you want to double-whammy high cholesterol and high blood pressure, take a second look at some of these fiber-rich grains.

Bran. There's nothing new about bran, just about the way people are eating it. It's making its way into everything from cereals to breads to snacks. And with good reason. Bran is the highest source of grain fiber you can get. It's actually the outer husk of grains like wheat, rye, oats, and rice, and it's usually separated from the flour after grinding. When the bran is removed, much of the fiber and nutrients go with it.

Breakfast cereals are probably the most popular source of bran. If you need some incentive to pour on the bran, take a look at the numbers when bran is compared with popular high-fiber vegetables:

- 1/3 cup unprocessed rice bran — 5.88 grams dietary fiber

- 1/3 cup raw oat bran — 4.77 grams dietary fiber

- 1 raw carrot — 2.16 grams dietary fiber

- 1/3 cup baked beans — 4.23 grams dietary fiber

Barley. Barley has been around since the Stone Age. Today it is used in everything from soups and breads to cereals and health drinks. Whole-grain barley is the most nutritious because it is the least processed. One cup contains a whopping 31 grams of fiber, along with loads of minerals. Pearl barley, which most people are familiar with, no longer has the bran, or outer husk, and is already steamed and polished. While it is still a healthy grain, many of the nutrients are removed during processing. One cup of pearl barley has about 6 grams of fiber. Quite a difference. On the other hand, if you bake, add some barley flour to your favorite recipe. One cup will give you near-ly 15 grams of fiber.

The heart benefits of barley have been well-proven. Researchers studying various forms of the grain, from flour to oil extract, found that barley can lower LDL cholesterol levels by as much as 9 percent. Even mixing barley into your every-day dishes, such as rice, makes a difference.

Oats. Oat bran, rolled oats, and whole-oat flour may be sporting a new heart-smart label: "May reduce the risk of heart disease." The FDA approved this claim for manufacturers of foods containing the soluble fiber from whole oats after the National Institutes of Health, the Centers for Disease Control and Prevention, and scientists at the FDA examined more than 30 studies. The general agreement was that the soluble fiber, known as beta glucan, found in oats is responsible for lowering cholesterol when eaten as part of a low-fat, low-cholesterol diet. Just 2 or 3 ounces a day were shown to make a difference.

Oat bran is perhaps the healthiest member of the oat fam-ily. It's high in potassium, phosphorus, and magnesium. Only one-third of a cup contains almost 5 grams of dietary fiber. Besides fighting high cholesterol, oat bran helps protect you from obesity and certain kinds of cancer.

Psyllium. If you picked up Metamucil and Kellogg's Bran Buds on your last trip to the supermarket, you bought the same ingredient in two different forms and perhaps for two dif-ferent reasons. Psyllium seed husk is technically an herb that acts as both an over-the-counter drug in Metamucil and other bulk laxatives, and most recently as an FDA-approved, heart-smart food additive to breakfast cereals.

A dozen medical studies found that eating psyllium-forti-fied cereal in addition to a low-fat diet reduces total cholesterol

and bad LDL cholesterol without affecting good HDL cholesterol. In fact, this combination seems to work better than just
following a low-fat diet. As little as three teaspoons (about 10
grams) of psyllium each day can lower your cholesterol. One
study showed this amount brought LDL levels down by 8 percent in just 8 weeks.

Other grain products you might want to try include:

- wild rice
- rice bran
- hominy
- semolina
- rice flour
- bulgur
- rye flour
- millet
- buckwheat groats

&. &. &.

You know the less refined your flour is, the more nutrients
it contains. A good way to test it is to run it through a sifter. If
most of it won't pass through, then you've got enough coarse,
unprocessed grain to be giving your heart a healthy benefit.

&. &.

Be creative — fiber doesn't have to be boring

If you're looking for something different to serve for dinner,
but still want a healthy dose of fiber, you've got more choices
than you probably thought. There are lots of grain and rice
alternatives from all over the world that are chock-full of fiber,
vitamins, and other nutrients — and they taste delicious, too.

Amaranth. A highly nutritious plant that has been grown
and eaten in Mexico for thousands of years. The Aztec and

Inca Indians harvested the seeds for cereal and flour, and perhaps even ate the greens, which are similar to spinach. Even though it has the unfortunate common name of "pigweed," amaranth is finally being taken seriously by scientists and nutritionists alike. Technically, it's not a grain but is used as one in cooking and baking. Amaranth is better for you than most grains. It contains more dietary fiber — one cup equals almost 30 grams, and it's particularly high in protein, calcium, iron, and the amino acid lysine.

Animal tests have shown amaranth to have some cholesterol-lowering abilities, and while there is no proof of this in humans, it is still a safe and nutritious product.

Quinoa. Although this food source has been overlooked by North Americans, it has been around for centuries. Quinoa was called "the mother grain" by the Incas as far back as the 14th century. Today, it has been described as the "supergrain of the future." High in protein, unsaturated fats, magnesium, iron, and potassium, quinoa has 10 grams of fiber per cup.

Triticale. A hybrid of wheat and rye, this grain combines the nutty flavor of wheat without the gluten. Triticale flour contains about 19 grams of fiber per cup.

Other cereal grains you might want to try are teff, spelt, couscous, and kamut. If you can't find these grains in your local supermarket, try health food stores, organic markets, mail-order houses, or Caribbean and Asian markets.

Swiss Muesli

1 1/2 cups rolled oats
1 1/2 cups water
2 cups shredded, unpeeled apples
1 1/2 cups (about 9 ounces) pitted prunes, whole or halved

2 tablespoons honey
2 tablespoons lemon juice
1/2 teaspoon cinnamon
fresh fruits (sliced banana, apple, pineapple, orange segments)
chopped almonds or pecans

Combine oats, water, shredded apples, prunes, honey, lemon juice, and cinnamon. Cover and refrigerate overnight.

In the morning, spoon some of the muesli into a cereal bowl. Top with your choice of fresh fruits and nuts. Serve with a dollop of plain yogurt or milk, if desired.

Muesli can be stored in a covered container in the refrigerator for several days.

Makes 6 servings

Per serving: 228 Calories (approximately); 2g Fat (0g from saturated fat) (8% calories from fat); 5g Protein; 51g Carbohydrate; 0mg Cholesterol; 5mg Sodium

This is an official 5 A Day Recipe. This recipe is provided by the California Prune Board.

Kiwifruit Bulgur Salad with Lemon Mint Dressing

1 cup bulgur wheat
1/2 cup sliced mushrooms
2 tablespoons butter or margarine
2 cups low sodium chicken broth
1/4 cup diagonally sliced green onions
1 cup finely shredded red cabbage
2 to 3 California kiwifruit (about 3 to 3 1/2 ounces each), pared and sliced

1 cooked chicken breast (10 to 12 ounces) boned, skinned and sliced, or 10 to 12 ounces cooked whitefish, cut into serving-sized pieces

Lemon Mint Dressing:

6 tablespoons lemon juice
2 tablespoons vegetable oil
4 teaspoons honey
2 teaspoons grated lemon peel
2 teaspoons fresh minced mint leaves (one teaspoon dried crushed mint can be substituted).

Combine dressing ingredients and mix well. Makes about 1/2 cup.

Sauté bulgur and mushrooms in butter until golden. Add chicken broth, cover, and bring to boil. Reduce heat and simmer 15 minutes. Cool.

Toss with green onions and 1/4 cup Lemon Mint Dressing.

Arrange bulgur, cabbage, and kiwifruit on plates with sliced chicken or fish. Drizzle with remaining Lemon Mint Dressing.

Makes 4 servings

Per serving: 406 Calories; 18g Fat (3.5g from saturated fat)(38% calories from fat); 23g Protein; 46g Carbohydrate; 36mg Cholesterol; 374mg Sodium

Reprinted with permission from the California Kiwifruit Commission. This salad can be served as a side dish with light meat, such as chicken or fish, or can be eaten alone.

Chocolate

Secret ingredient protects your arteries

Theobroma, the botanical name for cocoa beans, means "food of the gods." And if you're a chocolate lover, you couldn't agree more. There's something about the sweet, creamy taste of chocolate that is truly divine. So what could be even more heavenly? If your doctor said your favorite chocolate snack was good for your heart.

This may not be such a far-fetched idea. Scientists have discovered chemical properties in chocolate that could lower your cholesterol and cut your risk of heart disease.

It all begins with compounds called flavonoid phenolics, or phenols, found in chocolate and other foods, like apples, onions, tea, and wine. Research has proven that phenols reduce your risk of blood clots and act as antioxidants to keep LDL cholesterol from damaging your arteries. These are two important risk factors for heart disease.

You've probably heard of the heart benefits you can get from drinking a little red wine. It's because the phenols in the wine keep bad cholesterol from joining with oxygen and building up on your artery walls by as much as 65 percent. In the following chart, you can see how the phenols in chocolate compare to those in red wine.

Source	Serving size	Phenols (mg)
hot chocolate	1 cup (2 tablespoons cocoa)	146
milk chocolate	1.5 ounces	205
red wine	5 ounces	210

Some researchers are convinced of the protective effects of phenols. They say including a moderate amount of chocolate in a healthy diet could help guard against atherosclerosis. One study even tested a milk chocolate bar against a high-carbohydrate daily snack on men already eating a healthy, low-fat diet. Researchers found no difference in cholesterol levels between the two groups.

However, eating a piece of chocolate today won't save your heart next year, or even next week. The positive cholesterol effects don't last more than a couple of hours.

Don't be fooled into thinking you can indulge in as much chocolate as your heart desires. Chocolate is still about one-third saturated fat and is loaded with calories. Sticking to a low-fat diet, full of fruits, vegetables, and grains, is a much better way to get those important antioxidants.

🐜 🐜 🐜

What about caffeine?

When choosing your source of flavonoids, keep in mind that chocolate contains much less caffeine than coffee, black tea, or even green tea.

🐜 🐜

Consider cocoa butter a good saturated fat

The next time you're reading chocolate labels, look for the ingredient cocoa butter, the heart of true chocolate flavor. Cocoa butter is what remains inside the cocoa bean after several processing and drying steps. It has unique properties that allow chocolate to be mixed, formed, hardened, and melted. But from a health standpoint, cocoa butter is the good guy of saturated fats. In fact, human and animal tests have shown that cocoa butter causes less damage to arteries than other saturated fats.

That's because it is mostly made up of two specific fatty acids — stearic and oleic acid. Although these are saturated fatty acids, they do not affect cholesterol the way other saturated fats do. In fact, there is strong evidence that neither one raises cholesterol at all.

Buying tips for the healthiest chocolate

Unfortunately, all chocolate is not created equal. There are a few differences you should know about when shopping for your chocolate treat.

The darker your chocolate, like bittersweet or milk chocolate, the more phenols it contains. White chocolate, although high in cocoa butter, contains no phenols.

And although some of the finer chocolates contain a hefty amount of cocoa butter, most of the popular candy bars and chocolate sweets in your grocery store contain very little. Instead, they're full of cream and other forms of butterfat that give a rich taste but none of the good fats, like stearic or oleic fatty acid.

HERSHEY's 50% Reduced Fat Chocolatey Chip Cookies

2 1/4 cups all-purpose flour
1 teaspoon baking soda
1/2 teaspoon salt
1/2 cup margarine/butter blend
3/4 cup granulated sugar
3/4 cup packed light brown sugar
1 teaspoon vanilla extract
2 eggs
2 cups HERSHEY's reduced fat semisweet baking chips (12 ounce package)

Heat oven to 375 degrees F. Stir together flour, baking soda, and salt. In large bowl, beat spread, granulated sugar, brown sugar, and vanilla with electric mixer until creamy. Add eggs; beat well. Gradually add flour mixture, beating well. Stir in chips. Drop by rounded teaspoonfuls onto greased cookie sheet.

Bake 8 to 10 minutes or until lightly browned. Cool slightly; remove from cookie sheet to wire rack.

Variations:

Chewy Cookies: Add 1 to 2 tablespoons unsweetened apple-sauce to egg mixture.

Chocolate Chocolatey Chip Cookies: Add 1/3 cup HERSHEY's Cocoa to flour mixture; follow directions above for mixing and baking.

Pan recipe: Spray 15-1/2x10-1/2x1-inch jelly-roll pan with vegetable cooking spray; spread batter into pan. Bake at 375 degrees F. 18 to 20 minutes or until lightly browned. Cool completely; cut into bars.

Makes 5 dozen cookies or about 60 bars

Per serving: 77 Calories; 3g Fat (2g from saturated fat) (32% calories from fat); 1g Protein; 11g Carbohydrate; 8mg Cholesterol; 60mg Sodium

HERSHEY's is a registered trademark. Recipe courtesy of the Hershey Kitchens, and reprinted with permission of Hershey Foods Corporation. © Hershey Foods Corporation

Chromium

Miracle mineral fortifies your arteries

Although you only need small amounts of chromium, most people don't get enough. One study found that a group of people with heart disease had an average chromium level 41 percent lower than a group of people without heart disease.

Chromium is a trace mineral that helps your body produce and use insulin. Insulin transports glucose, also known as blood sugar, out of your blood and into your body's cells. There it's converted into energy. By helping your body maintain a steady supply of insulin, chromium helps keep glucose moving out of your blood at a steady rate. This prevents your blood sugar from going too high, as in diabetes, or too low, as in hypoglycemia.

Studies show chromium may help fight heart disease in several ways. Your body's main source of energy is glucose, but if it can't use glucose effectively, it has to find another energy source — fat. When your body uses fat as an energy source, some of the byproducts of the process are made into cholesterol. That could result in heart disease, and it may be one reason diabetics are much more likely to develop heart disease than people who don't have diabetes.

Animal studies suggest chromium can help counteract the effects of a high-sugar or high-cholesterol diet. Rats fed a high-sugar, chromium-deficient diet had a shocking buildup of fat in their arteries. When the rats got the same high-sugar diet with a chromium supplement, their cholesterol levels went down significantly, and they had less fat buildup in their arteries. Some studies on humans have supported those findings.

In one study, people with heart disease who took chromium chloride supplements raised their levels of good HDL cholesterol by about 10 points and also improved their triglyceride levels.

Chromium may also be helpful for people taking beta blockers. Although beta blockers are effective in lowering blood pressure, they can also lower levels of HDL cholesterol. One study found that men who were taking beta blockers were able to raise their HDL levels by taking 600 micrograms (mcg) of chromium a day.

Many foods contain chromium but much of it is lost when foods are processed. If you eat a lot of prepackaged, highly processed foods, you probably aren't getting enough.

Although there is no RDA for chromium, the Estimated Safe and Adequate Daily Dietary Intake for healthy adults is 50 to 200 mcg. You can increase your level of chromium naturally by eating more fresh, unprocessed foods and limiting your sugar intake. Foods that are good sources of chromium include:

asparagus	fresh fruit, especially apples with skin
beef	liver
brewer's yeast	mushrooms
chicken	nuts
dairy products	potatoes with skin
eggs	prunes
fish and seafood	whole-grain products

Chromium is difficult for your body to absorb so most supplements combine it with another substance, like picolinate, which helps it get into your cells. You can buy chromium supplements, but if you're taking a multi-vitamin, check the label. It may already be in there.

Although chromium appears to be fairly safe, use good judgment when taking supplements. One study found that chromium picolinate damaged the chromosomes in the ovary cells of hamsters, although the rodents received a dose several thousand times higher than the typical supplement taken by humans. Chromium nicotinate didn't have the same effect.

There have also been a few reports of toxicity, usually due to consuming very large quantities of chromium, which resulted in liver and kidney damage and increased rates of cancer.

If you're diabetic, talk with your doctor before taking any supplement.

The chromium-weight loss controversy continues

If you look in your drugstore for chromium supplements, chances are you'll find them with the weight loss aids. Many people have longed for a quick, easy way to lose fat and gain muscle, and early studies indicated that chromium might be the answer.

Since chromium helps your muscles use sugar, some researchers thought it would help those muscles "bulk up" and burn fat faster. The first studies looked encouraging. Athletes who took chromium picolinate supplements were able to lose more fat and gain more lean body mass than those who took a placebo. Several other studies, however, found that chromium supplements did not help people lose weight.

Results of another recent study were more positive. People who took 400 mcg of chromium picolinate for 90 days lost an average of 6.2 pounds, while people who took a placebo only lost 3.4 pounds.

Why the mixed results? It could be the way the studies were designed, or it could be that chromium affects different people in different ways. At any rate, the chromium-weight loss controversy is far from over.

If you want to take chromium supplements to help your weight loss efforts, it probably won't hurt, since most people are deficient in the mineral anyway. Just don't overdo it. And remember, so far the only surefire way to lose weight is to burn more calories than you take in.

Coenzyme Q10

Halt heart disease with high-energy enzyme

Coenzyme Q10 is one of a thousand tiny elements necessary for life. It's produced naturally in your body, but in order to produce it, your body needs vitamins C, B2, B3, B6, and folic acid. Without these building blocks, you can't make CoQ10.

This multi-talented enzyme is present in every cell of your body and works in each cell to produce energy. Without energy, your cells would die.

CoQ10 also provides plenty of antioxidant protection, which prevents cell damage. It may also help regenerate another antioxidant, vitamin E, allowing it to function as an antioxidant over and over.

Numerous studies have found that CoQ10 improves heart function, even restoring normal function to hearts already damaged by disease.

The most exciting studies on CoQ10 have involved its effect on people with congestive heart failure. Heart failure doesn't mean your heart stops, as it does in cardiac arrest. It just means your heart can't pump enough blood to supply all the parts of your body. Your body tries to compensate for your heart's deficiency by retaining salt and water, forcing your blood volume to increase. This can result in a buildup of fluid in your lungs, which can cause swelling in your legs or pneumonia.

The cells of your heart contain high levels of CoQ10, probably because those cells require so much energy. People with congestive heart failure, however, have CoQ10 levels lower than normal. In fact, the lower the CoQ10 levels, the more severe the heart disease, and vice versa.

Several studies have found that CoQ10 supplements improved heart function, allowed the heart to pump more blood, and decreased heart disease symptoms like breathlessness, fatigue, and chest pain. In some cases, the size and function of the heart returned to normal on CoQ10 alone.

Are supplements right for you?

Although there is no recommended dietary allowance (RDA) for CoQ10, too little of this enzyme can cause many health problems, including a depressed immune system, high blood pressure, obesity, heart disease, and a general lack of energy.

You can become deficient in CoQ10 in four ways:

- **Diet.** When you don't get enough vitamin C and B vitamins in your diet, your body can't produce CoQ10.

- **Getting older.** The natural aging process slows down your CoQ10 factory.

- **Disease.** Your body demands more if you are battling a disease.

- **Genetics.** A genetic defect prevents your body from making it.

A CoQ10 deficiency can't be fixed by taking a drug. If your body isn't making enough, there are only two ways to get more — eating the right foods or taking supplements.

Most CoQ10 studies were done using supplements in doses from 30 to 200 milligrams (mg) per day. One of the leading researchers of CoQ10 recommends therapeutic doses of 120 to 160 mg a day for people with heart disease and doses of 10 to 30 mg a day for healthy people who want to increase their energy levels.

CoQ10 is available at health food stores. Because it is fat-soluble, you should buy an oil-based gel cap or take it with food containing fat. As with most supplements, it is better to take it with meals.

Very few side effects have been reported with CoQ10, even in high doses. However, if you are taking the blood thinner Coumadin, CoQ10 could make it ineffective and increase your risk of blood clots.

Certain cholesterol-lowering drugs, beta blockers, antidepressants, and tranquilizers can actually discourage your body from making CoQ10.

Talk with your doctor before taking CoQ10 supplements. If he thinks they might help you, work closely with him and ask him to monitor your progress.

🙢 🙢 🙢

How to get Coenzyme Q10 naturally

Good food sources include organ meats, such as heart (especially beef), kidney, and liver; sardines and mackerel; bran; sesame; spinach; beans; soy; and peanuts.

🙢 🙢

11 reasons to try CoQ10

✦ **Improves blood flow**. It decreases your blood's stickiness, which improves circulation and decreases your risk of blood clots.

- **Prevents artery damage.** CoQ10 may prevent LDL (bad) cholesterol from combining with oxygen and damaging the walls of your blood vessels, which often leads to hardening of the arteries.

- **Relieves symptoms.** CoQ10 can improve many of the symptoms of congestive heart failure.

- **Lowers blood pressure.** Some doctors think CoQ10 might help lower high blood pressure.

- **Fights fatigue.** In one study, all of the participants said their feelings of tiredness and their difficulty breathing improved after taking CoQ10.

- **Restores your heart.** CoQ10 can reduce the thickening of the wall in the left ventricle, the chamber of the heart that pumps oxygen-rich blood throughout the body.

- **Reduces need for drugs.** Some people are able to cut back on their traditional drug therapy because their symptoms improve.

- **Renews your outlook.** Most people suffering from congestive heart failure who have taken CoQ10 found their quality of life improved.

- **Keeps you out of the hospital.** Statistics show that if you suffer from congestive heart failure and take CoQ10 you are less likely to be hospitalized.

- **Enhances exercise.** Studies have found CoQ10 can help repair cell damage caused by exercise.

- **Clobbers cancer?** One study found that people with cancer may survive longer on CoQ10 therapy. Another study showed CoQ10 might protect cells from cancer-causing free radical damage.

Coffee

Filter out the facts and lower your cholesterol

Do you take it black or sweet? In a tiny Styrofoam cup or a mug big enough to float the Titanic? True coffee lovers will tell you it makes a difference. They will speak of roasting time and aromas, bean crops and flavor. But the only heart-smart question you need to ask is, "Is it filtered?"

There may still be some debate on the subject, but most experts agree that there is a heart-healthy difference between filtered and unfiltered coffee.

Coffee beans contain a compound called diterpene. Several studies have proven that cafestol and kahweol, two specific fats in diterpene, are responsible for raising cholesterol. These fats are drawn out of the coffee beans and into the coffee by the hot water used during the brewing process. If you consistently drink boiled or unfiltered coffee, like Scandinavian, cafetiere, French-press, or Turkish, you can raise your cholesterol level by as much as 10 percent. And that increases your risk of heart disease.

But using a paper filter, or even a gold-mesh filter, during brewing catches and removes these diterpenes from the coffee. Without the diterpenes, filter-brewed coffee, in moderate amounts, will not affect your cholesterol.

Rest easy if you prefer the instant or percolated varieties. They do not seem to have any effect on cholesterol levels.

☙ ☙ ☙

Caffeine quiz

Can caffeine harm your health? Test your caffeine knowledge by taking this quiz. The answers are found in this chapter.

1. Drinking instant or percolated coffee can raise your cholesterol level.

   True   False

2. If you have high blood pressure, drinking coffee before exercising could cause your blood pressure to go up.

   True   False

3. Caffeinated beverages can help stabilize blood pressure after a meal.

   True   False

4. Researchers say drinking coffee does not increase your risk of heart disease.

   True   False

5. Herbal beverages are always caffeine-free.

   True   False

☙ ☙

Coffee's effect on blood pressure — here's the latest scoop

Since the early 1900s, coffee has been accused of causing all sorts of health problems, including high blood pressure. But, according to the latest research, if you regularly drink coffee, you probably won't experience any change in your blood pressure.

If you don't drink coffee very often, you might notice a slight rise in your blood pressure, but it will return to normal as soon as the caffeine leaves your system. This change will be no more than you might experience after light exercise, such as climbing a flight of stairs.

If you have high blood pressure, don't drink coffee before exercising because it could cause your blood pressure to go up.

🐜 🐜 🐜

Home remedy cures after-dinner dizziness

Here's some good news for caffeine lovers. Did you know that caffeinated beverages can help stabilize blood pressure after meals?

It's common for older people to experience a drop in blood pressure after eating. The medical name for the condition is postprandial (after-meal) hypotension (low blood pressure). You may feel lightheaded and dizzy when you stand up, or like you are about to faint. You can experience these symptoms even if you have high blood pressure.

Studies of healthy older people show that drinking coffee or tea right after a meal can prevent this drop in blood pressure. Caffeinated beverages raise the blood pressure just enough to hold off this potentially dangerous condition.

Younger people also experience this drop in blood pressure after eating, but they can usually combat it by getting up from the dinner table and taking a walk. Exercise raises blood pressure enough to keep away symptoms. But the safest option for you, if you're an older person, is to drink a caffeinated beverage, then take a walk only after you feel stable on your feet.

Coffee found innocent of causing heart disease

If you're a coffee lover but you've been avoiding it because you're worried about heart disease, you now have a reason to celebrate. Researchers say drinking coffee does not increase your risk of heart disease.

A recent study of over 85,000 women found a strong correlation between coffee drinking and smoking. Among women who drank six or more cups of coffee a day, 58 percent were smokers. This connection between smoking and coffee drinking may account for previous findings that indicated coffee contributed to heart disease. However, after taking the smoking factor into account, even women who drank six or more cups of coffee a day did not have a higher risk of developing heart disease.

Although several studies, including the Framingham Heart Study, have found no link between coffee and heart disease, some people experience heart palpitations or an irregular heartbeat after drinking regular coffee. And experts say if you already have heart problems, don't mix coffee with alcohol. Each increases your heart rate and the combined effect is dangerous if you have a weak or damaged heart.

Beware of coffee alternatives that pack a caffeine punch

Their names are exotic, and they bring images of tropical forests and deep jungles. And while it is true that these caffeine-rich beverages were first discovered in countries of South

America and the Far East, you can now find them in many herbal stores and specialty shops.

Guarana. This is one herbal stimulant you should stay away from if you have heart problems. Its caffeine content gives your nervous system such an immediate boost it has earned the nickname "Zoom." Practically a national drink in South American countries like Brazil, you can find the powdered form of guarana in most large health food stores. But beware, guarana is likely to make your heart go pitter-patter.

Yerba mate. Call it Paraguay tea or just plain mate, but get ready for a jolt to your nervous system. If brewed in the traditional method, mate (pronounced mah-tay) can contain anywhere from 500 to 750 milligrams (mg) of caffeine (compared to 80 to 175 mg in a cup of coffee). In this country, mate is sold as an herbal stimulant.

Cacao beans. Do you love chocolate? Well you'd love it even more if you lived in Mexico a few hundred years ago. Back then, cacao beans were used as money. Pretty tough decision — eat it or spend it? Nowadays, these evergreen seeds give us cocoa and chocolate, both sources of caffeine.

Kola nuts. These add flavor and caffeine to cola drinks, herbal blends, and some medicines. In South America and Africa, where they are grown, the natives chew the nuts for quick energy and to ward off hunger.

Ease your caffeine jitters with chicory

Chicory is truly a valuable gift from Mother Nature. All parts, from top to bottom, can be used. The young leaves are cooked like spinach, and the roots can be boiled and eaten like parsnips. An older plant yields greens similar to celery. But perhaps you know chicory best as a coffee substitute.

For this purpose, the root is sliced, dried, roasted, and ground. This roasted chicory, or succory as it is also called, is then mixed with coffee or tea as an extender, or it can be prepared on its own.

The taste of roasted chicory has been described as both bitter and mellow, and it's especially popular in Louisiana where the coffee-chicory blend is called New Orleans or Creole coffee.

The medical profession is pleased with chicory's popularity since this herb counteracts the caffeine in coffee. In fact, chicory has a calming, even sedative effect. Animal tests have shown that it slows the heart, much like digitalis or quinidine. Egyptians have used it for years as a folk remedy for a rapid heartbeat.

So the next time you visit a coffee house, check the menu. If they offer a chicory or chicory-blend drink, give it a try. The Food and Drug Administration (FDA) has recognized it as a safe product that is easier on your heart and nervous system than regular coffee.

Answers to the quiz

1. **False. But if you consistently drink unfiltered or boiled coffee, you could raise your cholesterol by as much as 10 points.**
2. **True**
3. **True**
4. **True**
5. **False. Some herbal beverages have more caffeine than coffee.**

Eating Out

How to order a meal your heart will love

Dinner with friends, carry-out on busy nights, or lunch from the drive-thru. Eating out is fun, easy, and sometimes it's necessary. But in order to keep your stomach and your heart happy, you must learn what foods to avoid once you leave home.

With portions becoming larger and larger, the problem is not only what you eat, but how much. You'll see words like "deluxe," "giant," and "jumbo" screaming from menus. That means bigger hamburgers with more artery-clogging meat, king-size servings of french fries with more saturated fat, and monster buckets of movie popcorn loaded with trans fatty acids. Consider sharing with a friend or ordering half-size portions, and don't be shy about asking for a doggie-bag.

When ordering from a restaurant menu, look for "light" or "healthy" selections. Many restaurants offer grilled or steamed fish or chicken and steamed vegetables. If your restaurant doesn't offer light choices, ask your waiter if you can get a healthier version of your order. If the dish is cooked in butter, see if it can be prepared with lemon or wine instead. Choose your side dishes carefully. Know which substitutions are healthier for your heart and ask for them. Most restaurants are happy to accommodate. The more you bring a need for healthy selections to the attention of the management, the more likely they are to make these choices a part of their regular menu.

What you do while you're waiting for your "real" food to come can be deadly. Some restaurants put out complimentary bowls of salty or deep-fried snacks, or you can order from a mouthwatering selection of appetizers. Unfortunately, most of these are also fried and come with fatty dips, sauces, and dressings. Stick to fruit, raw vegetables, or steamed seafood as starters.

If you're going to survive in today's world of dining, you'll need to learn some salad bar savvy. Don't load up your plate thinking that just because it's salad it must be healthy. Mayonnaise-based salads, like macaroni and potato salad, are overflowing with fat. Toppings like bacon bits, seeds, nuts, hard-boiled eggs, cheese, and croutons add fat, calories, and sodium. Even marinated vegetables are usually chock-full of oil and salt.

Your best bet is to eat your fill of fresh, raw fruits and vegetables. Pick the darkest green lettuce you can — it's healthier. And measure out the dressing with care. Creamy ones naturally have more fat. Even one tablespoon of regular Italian dressing has 7 grams of fat.

Remember, it's your total diet that's important. Splurging on a meal every so often will not make a big difference in your cholesterol levels or overall heart health. Just make sure you balance out a high-fat meal with more sensible eating the rest of the day.

Here are more healthy tips for your dining pleasure:

Sauce it on the side. Ask for gravy, dressings, and sauces to be served separately. Then use sparingly, especially if it isn't a light version.

Hold the cheese. Leave it off everything you can. It's full of saturated fat.

Go for the greens. Order salad instead of soup as a side dish or starter. Many soups are full of cream, cheese, or salt. If you find a bean-based soup on the menu, give it a try, and you'll be slurping up an added dose of fiber.

Select a spud. For less salt, order a baked potato instead of rice and add a sprinkle of chives and pepper for great flavor. Stay away from the loaded version, the one stuffed with cheese, bacon bits, sour cream, and butter.

Cook it right. Anything stir-fried is better than old stand-bys like lasagna or meat loaf. But broiled, roasted, steamed, or poached entrees are even better.

End with sweet success. Try fruit or sorbet for dessert instead of cakes, pies, cobblers, and ice cream.

Seek and ye shall find cholesterol-fighting fast food

Many fast food chains offer meals lower in saturated fat, calories, and cholesterol than those you would get at a popular dinner house restaurant. A regular hamburger at a restaurant can have twice as much fat as one from the drive-thru simply because it's bigger. Extra meat, extra cheese, and extra sauce only mean extra artery-clogging fat. But watch out for the hidden sodium in fast food fare. Did you know a milkshake has more sodium than a regular order of french fries?

Although you keep hearing that fish and chicken are better for you than red meat, even the leanest piece of chicken can be ruined by dipping it into batter and deep-frying. Given the choice, a plain hamburger is healthier.

If you must have a traditional side dish, choose the lesser of two evils — french fries over onion rings. The fries have less fat, calories, and salt. One order of onion rings has more saturated fat than most entrees.

Here are some other good fast food choices:

- wraps, pitas, or tortilla sandwiches, but hold the cheese and dressings

- pizzas with vegetarian toppings and half the cheese

- a lean roast beef sandwich

Don't let breakfast be your arteries' worst nightmare

Breakfast bars and buffets are a weekend tradition for many people. Unfortunately, most breakfast fare is high in cholesterol, saturated fat, sodium, and calories.

If you want to start the day right, order cereal, either hot or cold, preferably with 1 percent or skim milk. Add juice; a bagel, English muffin, or toast without butter; and fruit, and you're on your way to a healthy day.

If you decide you've just got to have an omelette, forget the cheese and make it strictly vegetarian. If you can, order it made with an egg substitute or just egg whites.

Sausage is the worst breakfast side dish you can order. If you must have a breakfast meat, Canadian bacon may be your best choice.

If you're craving pancakes and syrup, skip the butter and pour on low-calorie syrup. You'll never taste the difference. Low-calorie syrup has half the calories of regular syrup. A very smart trade-off.

A Belgian waffle is higher in saturated fat than pancakes or biscuits and gravy. If you just can't deny yourself, top it with fresh fruit and leave off the whipped cream.

Croissants, biscuits, doughnuts, and pastries are deadly on your arteries. Go for almost any other type of bread, but try to make it whole-grain.

Mama Mia! Choose Italian dishes wisely

Pasta is a healthy choice for a restaurant meal, just watch out for the sauce. Cream and cheese-based sauces, like Alfredo and carbonara, are the worst. Marinara, wine, mushroom, and clam sauces are better. Many Italian favorites like cheese manicotti, cannelloni, and ravioli are stuffed with saturated fat.

Lasagna and Fettuccini Alfredo are probably the two fattiest dishes you can order, while pasta primavera is a great heart-healthy choice.

Here are three other common Italian foods full of hidden, heart-breaking danger:

Parmesan cheese. Add 1 gram of saturated fat for every tablespoon you sprinkle on.

Eggplant parmigiana. This innocent-looking vegetarian dish is fried in oil.

Garlic bread. It's loaded with saturated fat and salt.

Smart eating south of the border

You may think Mexican food has got to be healthy. Chicken, beans, and tortillas sound pretty safe, but don't forget all that cheese and sour cream. Even a healthy dish like rice and beans can become your arteries' worst nightmare with the extra salt, lard, bacon, and cheese most restaurants add for flavor. The saturated fat content goes off the scale.

One way to lower the fat is to order your food without guacamole, cheese, and sour cream toppings. Instead spoon salsa over your meal for lots of low-fat flavor. Your safest south-of-the-border bets are chicken fajitas, tacos, or burritos.

Here are two popular Mexican dishes that will make your heart pound with fear:

Chimichangas. These are deep-fried in oil, which spells clogged arteries for you. And remember ... tortilla chips are deep-fried, too.

Taco salads. Because of the fried shell, ground beef, sour cream, cheese, and guacamole, they can contain over 1,000 calories and half a day's supply of fat.

5 ways to chop fat and sodium from Chinese food

A meal at your favorite Chinese restaurant can be both fun and exotic. Unfortunately, it can also be full of fat, salt, and calories. That's because traditional, healthy, Asian cooking has been changed over the years to accommodate Western tastes.

But you can still get a Chinese meal your heart will love without traveling to the other side of the world. Just keep these tips in mind:

- Make steamed rice the basis of your meal. Order lots of it and pile it on your plate first.

- Divide up your entrees. Set aside half to take home for later. Mix the other half with an order of extra steamed vegetables.

- Take small portions of your entree and mix with the rice. Leave as much sauce behind as possible.

- Hold off on the beef and pork dishes. Instead, choose vegetables, chicken, or seafood.

- Ask for low-sodium soy sauce.

For more healthy Chinese eating tips, see the *Eating plans* chapter.

Reel in a low-fat catch of the day

Almost any fish entree is going to be healthier than a red meat choice. That is, unless it is breaded, fried, cream-sauced, or stuffed. But you can't go wrong if you order your fish broiled, baked, blackened, grilled, or steamed. Be sure and throw back the tartar sauce. One tablespoon has 182 milligrams (mg) of sodium and 8 grams of fat.

Ordering a meal of lobster, clams, crab, or shrimp will give you about zero grams of saturated fat. And if you pair it up with a plain baked potato, rolls, and a salad with lemon juice or vinegar, you've got just about the healthiest meal you can get at a restaurant — low in calories, fat, and sodium.

Fried platters are simply saturated fat on a plate. More than one-third of your fried fish entree is breading or batter, with fried clams having the worst ratio of fish to breading. Many seafood restaurants still use solid shortening for frying. Find out if your favorite shrimp shack uses vegetable oil. If not, let them know you're concerned, and perhaps they'll change their policy.

8 ways to build a winning sandwich

Who would have thought the innocent little sandwich could turn out to be not so innocent after all. One reason is that it's not so little. Most sandwich shops pile on anywhere from 5 ounces to half a pound of filling. That's more than double the recommended serving amount.

Perhaps the worst thing sandwich shops can do is overlook all the low-fat, low-sodium, light ingredients they could be using. Instead, you'll probably get full-fat cheese and mayo, regular sodium ham, and regular fat dressings.

Here are some tips that will help you build a sandwich to make your heart proud.

Surrender the mayo. Even though it's been a part of sandwiches since man first slapped together two pieces of bread, regular mayonnaise is full of saturated fat — the kind that clogs arteries. Better choices are fat-free or low-fat mayo, mustard, or vinegar for zing. Even ketchup is a healthier choice.

Go easy with the sides. Watch out for potato chips, pickles, cole slaw, and potato salad. Add any of these and your fat and sodium intake will go through the roof. Try carrot or celery sticks for a little crunchy fun, or go with a green side salad.

Gobble down turkey. Turkey is your healthiest meat filling but ask for a low-salt version. The more processed the meat, the more sodium and added fat. That means meats like corned beef, salami, bologna, and even ham are not as healthy as turkey, chicken, or lean roast beef.

Shun these salads. Watch out for the hidden fat in chicken, egg, and tuna salads. Besides the dressing mixed into the salad, many shops put mayo on the bread as well.

Eliminate the extras. Put a hold on the cheese, oil, salt, and bacon.

Gather a harvest of grains. Order your sandwich on whole wheat bread or rolls for an extra fiber boost.

Know the value of veggies. Almost anything that grows can be made into a sandwich. Try some unusual choices, like sprouts, but watch the fat by leaving off the cheese, avocado, and dressing.

Extinguish the grill. Grilled sandwiches like reubens, patty melts, and grilled cheese are slathered in saturated fat. If you love a bit of crunch, ask for your sandwich bread or bun toasted — but not buttered.

Guide to fast food eating

Selection	Saturated fat (grams)	Total fat (grams)	Calories	Sodium (mg)
Subway 6-inch Turkey Sub*	1	5	320	1,190
Arby's Light Roast Beef Deluxe	3	10	300	830
Wendy's Broccoli & Cheese Potato	3	14	470	470
Boston Market 1/4 Dark Chicken	3	10	210	320
Taco Bell Bean Burrito	4	12	380	1,140
Arby's Grilled Chicken Deluxe	4	20	430	850
Wendy's Chicken Caesar Pita	5	18	490	1,320
Subway 6-inch Tuna Sub*	5	32	540	890
Boston Market Meat Loaf & Tomato Sauce	8	18	370	1,170
McDonald's French Fries (large)	9	22	450	290
McDonald's Big Mac	10	31	560	1,070
Burger King Whopper	11	39	640	870

*Not including optional cheese, mayonnaise, or oil.

Eating Plans

Turn over a new leaf for your heart's sake

Billions of dollars are spent each year on heart surgeries, which sometimes provide only short-lived benefits and don't really increase your chances of living longer. What if you could prevent and treat heart disease cheaply and effectively, without stepping foot in a hospital? You can —simply by changing what you eat and adopting a healthy lifestyle.

Although your physical condition is a complex combination of heredity, environment, and lifestyle, healthy eating combined with sensible lifestyle changes can work wonders. It can even reverse severe artery damage.

Scrubbing clogged arteries clean

Would you like to cut down on the amount of plaque in your arteries? What about blood clots? Do you want to keep LDL cholesterol from joining with oxygen and hanging around in your bloodstream? And, of course, you want relaxed, free-flowing arteries. With the right diet, you can accomplish all of this — and more.

Before you read about some specific eating plans to beat heart disease, here are a few general guidelines for heart-healthy eating.

Reduce LDL cholesterol. Stock your pantry with soy products, legumes (peas and beans), garlic, and nuts. Eat foods rich in soluble fiber like oat bran, oatmeal, barley, and fruits and vegetables. Stay away from saturated fats found in animal and dairy products, such as meat, milk, butter, cheese, cream, egg yolks, and a few vegetable fats, like coconut oil, palm oil, and hydrogenated shortenings. Also avoid trans fatty acids. They are formed when margarines and other fats are hardened by a process called hydrogenation. Trans fatty acids are almost as bad for your arteries as saturated fat. You'll find them in hard margarines, fast foods, chips, and many baked goods. If you want to cut your "bad" fat intake in half, simply stop eating butter or margarine, fatty meats, and whole milk or 2 percent dairy products.

Dodge artery-clogging plaque. By adding monounsaturated fats, such as canola and olive oils, and fruits and vegetables to your diet, you can help keep LDL cholesterol from turning into artery-clogging plaque.

Stop blood clots. For the most benefit, eat more garlic and seafood and, if you drink, have a glass of red wine.

The U.S. Department of Agriculture and the U.S. Department of Health and Human Services have come up with their own guidelines:

- **Eat a variety of foods.** In order to get the right balance of nutrients, eat foods from all food groups. They each offer something unique and necessary to good health.

- **Maintain a healthy weight.** A major risk factor for heart disease is excess weight. A good eating plan full of low-fat, whole-grain foods will keep the pounds off and your heart healthy.

- **Trim the fat.** Keep total fat, saturated fat, and cholesterol intake low.

- **Load up on plant foods.** By eating plenty of vegetables, fruits, and grain products, you'll be giving your body a natural source of vitamins, minerals, and cholesterol-busting antioxidants.

- **Watch the sweets.** Use table sugar and sugared products in moderation.

- **Lower your salt.** Whether it comes out of a shaker or shows up in processed foods, salt should be a small part of your daily diet.

- **Limit the alcohol.** Drink only in moderation. Most experts agree that "one drink" equals a 12-ounce bottle of beer, a 4-ounce glass of wine, or a 1 1/2-ounce shot of 80-proof spirits. Consuming one or two of these drinks a day is usually considered moderate drinking.

There are lots of small, easy changes you can make in your daily eating habits that will mean big heart benefits. Be patient and don't give up. It could take your body several months to adjust to these changes in diet. If you don't see improvements after that amount of time, talk to your doctor.

Understanding food label fast talk

Now that you've decided to eat for a healthy heart, you've got to go shopping. You'll probably feel overwhelmed by the variety of packaged foods, all claiming to be low-fat, free, and light. And what about those percentages? Just because you're selecting an oat cereal doesn't mean it isn't loaded with fat, salt, or sugar. To choose the best product, you must take time to read labels.

Nutrition Facts label. First, read the Nutrition Facts label. On these new labels, you'll find serving size, calories, car-

bohydrates, fiber, protein, vitamins and minerals, fat, cholesterol, and sodium.

Nutrition Facts

Serving Size 1 cup (228g)
Servings Per Container 2

Amount Per Serving

Calories 260   Calories from Fat 120

	% Daily Value*
Total Fat 13g	**20%**
Saturated Fat 5g	**25%**
Trans Fat 2g	
Cholesterol 30mg	**10%**
Sodium 660mg	**28%**
Total Carbohydrate 31g	**10%**
Dietary Fiber 0g	**0%**
Sugars 5g	
Protein 5g	

Vitamin A 4%	•	Vitamin C 2%
Calcium 15%	•	Iron 4%

*Percent Daily Values are based on a 2,000 calorie diet.
Your Daily Values may be higher or lower depending on
your calorie needs:

	Calories:	2,000	2,500
Total Fat	Less than	65g	80g
Sat Fat	Less than	20g	25g
Cholesterol	Less than	300mg	300mg
Sodium	Less than	2,400mg	2,400mg
Total Carbohydrate		300g	375g
Dietary Fiber		25g	30g

Calories per gram:
Fat 9   •   Carbohydrate 4   •   Protein 4

The % Daily Value is perhaps the most helpful number
since very few people can remember the recommended
amounts. This tells you how much of a nutrient you'll be

getting in a serving of that particular food. It is based on a 2,000 calorie a day diet. If a food contains 5 percent or less of the Daily Value for a nutrient, it's not a high source of that nutrient. That's good for things like cholesterol and saturated fat, but you want higher percentages for vitamins and minerals.

Product claims. Next, arm yourself with a grasp of a few basic terms, and you'll never again be at the mercy of food label fast talk. The language has been standardized by the government, which means certain terms mean very specific things.

Fat free	Less than 0.5 gram of fat per serving
Low-fat	No more than 3 grams of fat per serving
Lean	Less than 10 grams of fat, 4 grams of saturated fat, and 95 milligrams (mg) of cholesterol per serving
Light (Lite)	One-third less calories or no more than half the fat of the higher-calorie, higher-fat version; or no more than half the sodium of the higher-sodium version
Reduced calorie	At least 25 percent fewer calories per serving than the regular version
Sugar-free	Less than 0.5 gram of sugar per serving
Good source of calcium	At least 100 mg of calcium per serving
High-protein	At least 10 grams of high-quality protein
Low-cholesterol	Less than 20 mg of cholesterol and no more than 2 grams of saturated fat per serving

In addition, if a product claims to be good for your heart, it must be low in total fat, saturated fat, and cholesterol. To make a health claim about high blood pressure, the product must be low in sodium.

Pick an eating plan you can stick to

To make it easier for you to take that first step toward better heart health, here are five easy-to-follow eating plans that have hard medical evidence to back up their heart-saving claims.

The Asian diet — humble eating for a healthy heart

It took the largest study of its kind, but the results are undeniable. If you want to live longer and healthier, eat like an Asian peasant.

Researchers have known for some time that people living in countries like China, Japan, Thailand, India, Korea, and Indonesia have a lower risk of cancer, obesity, and heart disease. They just never had the hard evidence to tell them why. Now they do.

In a Chinese diet study, called the China-Cornell-Oxford Diet and Health Project, researchers have been collecting information on the eating habits of over 10,000 Chinese since 1983. They've found that poor, rural Asians eat a humble, traditional diet — full of soyfoods and high-fiber grains and vegetables, with few animal products. This, they say, is the reason for their good health. Cholesterol levels are low, so low in fact that their average high cholesterol is still about equal to the lowest range in the United States. And only an average of 15 percent of deaths in Asia are due to heart disease, compared with more than 40 percent in the United States.

The super heart-saving Asian diet has won the approval of many nutrition experts because it emphasizes plant-based, rather than animal-based, foods. Following this type of eating pattern may be your path to sound health and a long life.

The Asian food pyramid

Here are the basic groups that make up the Asian food pyramid. There are many ways to include these foods in your everyday eating without having to give up your own traditions. On the other hand, if you're tired of the same old meat and potatoes routine, why not buy a Chinese cookbook and learn the art of stir-frying.

You can read more heart-saving information about many of these foods in their separate chapters.

Grains. According to the Asian pyramid, most of your diet should consist of unrefined rice, wheat, millet, corn, barley, and other grains. Other dishes are generally eaten alongside, but only in small amounts, to add variety and zest.

Although white rice is widely eaten in Eastern countries, it is less polished than what you probably buy. That means it still has more of the fiber-rich outer layers and is, therefore, healthier all-around. Look for unpolished rice the next time you go shopping. And while you're being adventurous, pick up some basmati, jasmine, or brown rice. They are full of flavor, fragrance, and fiber.

Vegetables. Whether from the land or the sea, vegetables play a big part in the everyday Asian diet. Some that you may find in traditional Asian recipes are bok choy, Chinese mustard greens, amaranth, water spinach, water chestnuts, bamboo shoots, lotus root, and bitter melon.

If these aren't in your local grocery store or just don't seem like your cup of tea, don't despair. Vegetables like broccoli, spinach, celery, carrots, and peppers are easily adapted to traditional Asian recipes. Throw in some sprouts and spices, and you'll think you're in the Land of the Rising Sun.

Soy. Whether they're made into milk, tofu, paste, noodles, or sheets, soybeans are an important and versatile part of the Asian diet. Rich in fiber and phytoestrogens, soybeans are a proven ally against heart disease and cancer.

Since animal products are a small part of the Asian diet, and vitamin B12 is only found in animal products, you might not be getting enough of this important vitamin. To solve this problem, buy vitamin B12-fortified soy products.

Unfortunately, the soy picture is not all rosy. Many experts are concerned about the connection between soy and forgetfulness discovered several years ago. The research suggests soy makes your brain age faster — the more soy you eat, the greater your memory and learning difficulties and the greater your risk of developing senility. While you don't have to avoid soy altogether, talk to your doctor about keeping to moderate amounts.

Legumes. When you cut out animal products, you may worry about getting enough protein. A great vegetarian substitute is the small but mighty, protein-rich legume. Peas and beans are a huge source of fiber. They should be part of at least one meal a day. Besides soybeans, other legumes you can try for an authentic Asian taste are mung beans, chickpeas, and lentils.

Nuts and seeds. Almonds, cashews, walnuts, pine nuts, and chestnuts are all popular ingredients in Asian cooking. Many are crushed and mixed with water to form nut milk, which is then used in sauces, desserts, and dressings. Try to get about a handful of nuts or seeds every day.

Fats and oils. Small amounts of peanut, golden sesame, soy, and corn oils may be eaten daily.

Seafood. Although it's often more expensive than chicken or red meat, fish is worth the extra pennies. It's full of healthy omega-3 fatty acids and protein, but low in cholesterol. People living in places where eating fish is part of the culture have much lower cholesterol levels. To make fish go further in your budget, follow the Asian way and chunk it up in your favorite stir-fry or soup.

Meat. Compared with a Western diet, the traditional Chinese diet has much less protein. And what protein the Chinese do eat generally comes from plant sources, not animals. To help keep your arteries healthy, some experts recommend eating red meat only once a month and cutting back on poultry and eggs — no more than an average serving each week.

Herbs. No eating plan would be complete without the herbs and spices unique to that culture. Many not only add flavor and spice to the food, but some, like garlic, turmeric, and fenugreek, provide powerful heart protection, too.

Sweets. If you want to follow the Asian diet, you must cut back on sugar and sweets. In Asia, fresh fruits, not sweets, are served for dessert.

🐜 🐜 🐜

Restaurant eating that's good for your heart

Traditional Oriental food is not necessarily what you'll get at your local Chinese restaurant. Western tastes call for more meat, fewer vegetables, lots of fat and deep-frying, and so much sodium you better take your blood pressure medicine before you even sit down. And if you're visiting a Thai restaurant, beware of dishes made with coconut oil or milk. Unless you share with several friends, you'll be getting an unhealthy dose of saturated fat.

Choose tofu dishes, soups, stir-fried meats without breading, and vegetarian entrees; load up on steamed rice and other grains; and go easy with the soy sauce.

🐜 🐜

The DASH diet —
a natural way to lower blood pressure

Don't ignore high blood pressure. It increases your risk for heart disease and stroke. But you can bring down blood pressure without medication by simply changing what you eat. The best news is you could see results in as little as two weeks.

Research for the DASH (Dietary Approaches to Stop Hypertension) diet was funded by the National Heart, Lung, and Blood Institute with support from the National Institutes of Health. They found that a diet high in grains, fruits, and vegetables and low in meats and fats significantly reduces blood pressure. Experts say lowering blood pressure by even a small amount across a population could cut down the amount of heart disease by 15 percent and stroke by almost 30 percent.

The diet recommends you eat eight servings of grains and up to 10 servings of fruits and vegetables every day. Most people eat less than half this amount. Studies show these foods help keep your arteries clear of fat deposits and your blood running smoothly.

It's important you also follow a healthy lifestyle — maintain a healthy weight, exercise regularly, eat foods low in salt, quit smoking, and use alcohol moderately, if at all. And don't stop taking any blood pressure medications without talking to your doctor first.

The second phase of the DASH study is called DASH2. It looks at how different levels of salt combined with test diets affect blood pressure. For this information and other news pertaining to the DASH diet, visit the official web site http://dash.bwh.harvard.edu/.

Tips on eating the DASH way

Grains. To get a major dose of energy and fiber, make whole-grain foods the bulk of your diet — seven to eight servings each day. And don't think just bread, include other grain products, like pitas, muffins, bagels, oatmeal, pasta, cereal, and rice. Just select whole-grain varieties. They are less refined and full of natural fiber.

Fruits and vegetables. There's nothing better for you than the wholesome products of Mother Nature. Fruits and vegetables are rich sources of magnesium, potassium, and fiber, which help lower blood pressure. There are dozens of ways, besides munching on them raw, to get the eight to 10 servings you need every day. Snack on them dried; drink juices; try new salad combinations for interest and variety; and serve fruits as a low-fat, low-calorie dessert.

Dairy. There is a place for dairy foods in the DASH diet, as long as you choose low-fat or nonfat products. Your body needs the calcium and protein you get from milk, yogurt, and cheese.

Meat, poultry, and fish. Unlike vegetarian eating plans, the DASH diet calls for up to 6 ounces of meat, chicken, or fish a day. The secret, though, is to treat it as one part of your entire meal, instead of the main part. In other words, center your meal around carbohydrates, such as pasta, rice, beans, or vegetables. Make sure you choose lean cuts, trim away as much fat or skin as you can, and cook it without oil.

Nuts, seeds, and legumes. For a healthy serving of protein, potassium, magnesium, and fiber, nothing fills the bill quite like legumes. At least four or five times a week make them a part of your main meal. If you're not a big fan of peas or beans, don't give up. You'll be surprised how easy it is to sneak them into your favorite recipes. They can really add an energy punch to soups, salads, and casseroles. Don't forget the nuts, either. A handful of peanuts, almonds, or sunflower seeds can be a great on-the-go snack.

The Mediterranean diet — the secret to a long life

The Greeks really know how to live it up. They eat crusty whole-grain breads, fresh fish, lush salads drenched with olive oil, and they drink wine in moderation. It seems this all adds up to a long and healthy life.

Years ago, researchers discovered that people living in Mediterranean countries live longer than people in other parts of the world and suffer from fewer chronic diseases.

Fewer people die from heart disease, even when their cholesterol levels are the same as those from other countries.

In an effort to find out why, an eating plan was developed, based on the culture and habits of several of these southern European countries. It became known as the Mediterranean diet. Researchers wanted to find out if a diet full of grains, fruits, vegetables, and olive oil and low in sweets, meat, and dairy foods could prevent heart disease.

To test this hypothesis, two groups of heart attack survivors were followed for more than two years. The group on the Mediterranean diet had an amazing 70 percent fewer deaths from heart-related causes.

The Mediterranean pyramid

The traditional Greek diet is high in monounsaturated fat (olive oil), high in complex carbohydrates (grains and legumes), high in fiber (fruits and vegetables), and low in saturated fat (animal and dairy products, like meat, milk, butter, cheese, cream, and egg yolks, and a few vegetable fats, such as coconut oil, palm oil, and hydrogenated vegetable shortenings). A low-fat, high-fiber diet, such as this, has been proven to reduce LDL cholesterol by almost 20 percent. In addition, natural antioxidants, like vitamin E, found in these foods will slow down, if not prevent, the development of atherosclerosis.

Plant foods. Plant foods rather than animal foods are the main part of the Mediterranean diet. You'll find most meals are made up of grains like couscous, pasta, polenta, rice, or bulgur and fresh vegetables. Legumes, such as chickpeas, are added to soups, stews, and salads as an important source of protein and fiber. Desserts are often fruits and nuts instead of cakes or cookies.

Olive oil. The Greeks consume large amounts of olive oil. This monounsaturated fat has been proven to lower LDL cholesterol and raise HDL cholesterol, which helps keep your arteries clear of fatty deposits and lowers your risk of heart attack. But remember olive oil should be used in place of saturated or hydrogenated fats and instead of other sources of calories. Otherwise you'll achieve no health benefits at all.

Less meat. Red meat plays only a minor role in the Mediterranean diet and is usually eaten just a couple of times a month. Fish and chicken are more common in Mediterranean meals, but they are usually not served more than a few times a week. Choose fish high in omega-3 fatty acids like herring, mackerel, salmon, and lake trout. These particularly help protect against heart disease.

Dairy. The preferred Greek dairy products are yogurt and feta cheese, but even these are used only sparingly. Since cheese from goats and sheep has a strong flavor, a little goes a long way. This helps cut down on the amount of saturated fat in your diet.

Wine. Moderate amounts of wine are a normal part of a Greek meal. For men this means two glasses of wine a day and one glass a day for women. Many studies suggest this amount reduces the risk of heart disease.

🐜 🐜 🐜

Save your heart and kick cancer, too

New research says following the Mediterranean diet may not only be good for your heart, it may protect against cancer, too. In a four-year follow-up study, scientists found that those following the Mediterranean diet had over 60 percent fewer deaths from cancer. They believe the large amounts of fiber, omega-3 fatty acids, and vitamin C, as well as less cholesterol and saturated fat, in the diet have something to do with this good news.

🐜 🐜

The Ornish program —
lifestyle changes can work a miracle

Want to lose weight without dieting, reverse heart disease without drugs or surgery, feel better than you ever have in your life, and get your insurance company to pay for it? Then Dr. Dean Ornish has the miracle you've been looking for. He is the author of *Dr. Dean Ornish's Program for Reversing Heart Disease*, a lifestyle program that advocates daily aerobic exercise; daily stress reduction; and a very low-fat, vegetarian diet. Ornish says if you limit the fats in your diet — particularly saturated fats — you'll be on your way to cleaner, freer-flowing arteries.

For many people, this program gives big results. It's been shown to decrease LDL levels by almost 40 percent. And within a short period of time, angina all but disappears. You can even reverse artery damage by making changes to your diet and lifestyle.

In one of the recent programs Ornish conducted, 82 percent of the participants experienced a significant reversal in their coronary artery disease within the first year — all without drugs or surgery.

What you eat more important than amount

If you've been diagnosed with heart disease or want to lose weight, Ornish recommends that no more than 10 percent of your calories come from fat. He also calls for the biggest chunk of your diet to be complex carbohydrates, with only about 20 percent of your calories from protein. In addition, he suggests you take in only 5 milligrams (mg) of cholesterol a day.

If all this sounds like too much math for you, don't worry. Ornish doesn't really say you need to constantly count calories or fat grams, you just need to realize that the type of food you eat is more important than the amount.

With that in mind, don't eat commercially prepared foods, eat whenever you feel hungry, eat until you are full, and stick to these guidelines.

Vegetarian. Eat complex carbohydrates or starches. Fruits, vegetables, grains, and legumes are natural forms of complex carbohydrates. These are high in fiber and fill you up without adding lots of calories.

Fat. Avoid all oils and stay away from high-fat foods, even vegetarian ones like avocados, olives, coconut, nuts, seeds, and cocoa concoctions. By eating mostly plant foods, you'll be cutting fat and cholesterol.

Animal products. With the exception of egg whites and one cup of nonfat yogurt or milk a day, for vitamin B12, you should avoid all animal products. By eating vegetables, grains, and legumes, you'll be getting calcium and protein without any cholesterol.

Alcohol. Limit alcohol to 2 ounces per day or less.

Caffeine. Try to avoid caffeine, which may worsen irregular heartbeats or provoke stress.

Sugar. Sugar, by itself, is not strongly linked to heart disease. It's just usually found in foods high in saturated fat and cholesterol. By avoiding one, you are avoiding the others.

Salt. Salt raises blood pressure in some people. If you are salt-sensitive, avoid it. If not, use salt in moderation.

Ornish recommends you follow his guidelines for at least three weeks. That's how long it takes to break bad habits and establish new, healthy habits.

The Step diets — eating to lower cholesterol

If you have high cholesterol, the National Institutes of Health has just the diet for you. Endorsed by the American Heart Association and the National Cholesterol Education

Program (NCEP), the Step diets help you conquer heart disease one step at a time.

The main purpose of these two eating plans is to reduce your LDL cholesterol. This cholesterol travels to the walls of your arteries where it eventually causes a fatty build-up. That means narrowed arteries, atherosclerosis, stroke, or heart attack. The higher your LDL, the greater your risk of heart disease. The best way to control this is to limit the amount of saturated fat you eat. And that's exactly what you'll do on a Step diet.

Although some experts say you can eliminate the need for cholesterol-lowering medication by following a healthy eating plan, you must also exercise regularly, stop smoking, and lose weight.

Step I diet. If you are not suffering from heart disease, but simply need to lower your cholesterol, the Step I diet may be for you. It lowers cholesterol by cutting saturated fat and balancing fiber and nutrients. The results may be modest, but for every cholesterol point you drop, you dramatically lower your risk of heart disease.

On the Step I diet you should eat:

- 8 to 10 percent of the day's total calories from saturated fat

- 30 percent or less of the day's total calories from fat

- less than 300 mg of cholesterol a day

- a controlled amount of calories to maintain a healthy weight

Step II diet. If you are at high risk for heart disease or you already have heart disease, your doctor might recommend the Step II diet. It might also help lower your cholesterol level if it didn't come down very much following Step I.

The guidelines for Step II are more strict. Generally, you're allowed less meat and eggs but more servings of unsaturated vegetable fats and oils. Studies have shown that following a diet such as this can lower your cholesterol from 5 to 20 percent. However, results may vary.

On the Step II diet you should eat:

- less than 7 percent of the day's total calories from saturated fat

- 30 percent or less of the day's total calories from fat

- less than 200 mg of cholesterol a day

- a controlled amount of calories to maintain a healthy weight

Both the Step I and II diets are based on percentages of the calories you eat. Since you could be taking in anywhere from 1,200 to 2,500 calories a day, the amount of fat and saturated fat grams varies. To make following the program easier, this chart has the percentages figured out for you. Remember 1 gram of fat equals 9 calories. You might find it helpful to discuss these numbers with a registered dietitian or nutritionist.

	Saturated fat grams per day				
Calories	**1,200**	**1,500**	**1,800**	**2,000**	**2,500**
Step I (9%)	12	15	18	20	25
Step II (6%)	8	10	12	13	17

	Total fat grams per day				
Calories	**1,200**	**1,500**	**1,800**	**2,000**	**2,500**
Step I (30%)	40	50	60	65	80
Step II (30%)	40	50	60	65	80

For more help choosing the right foods, read the new food labels. They list every nutrition fact you'll need to follow the Step I or Step II diet.

If you stick to one of these eating plans, you should see some results within a few weeks. Of course, your success will depend on several factors, but many people report an overall drop of 10 to 50 mg/dL in blood cholesterol levels.

Eating in STEP may save your heart

Meat, poultry, and fish. When buying meat, go for the leanest choice possible. Avoid marbled steaks and processed meats like bacon, hot dogs, and lunch meats; trim the fat; skin your chicken; and choose low-fat fish, such as cod. Studies show fish may be even better than chicken at keeping HDL cholesterol levels high. Stick to small portions — between 5 and 6 ounces a day. If you don't want to weigh your food, keep in mind that 3 ounces of meat is about the size of a deck of cards.

Dairy. Avoid whole and 2 percent milk, cheese, and ice cream. Unless you're picking up the low-fat or nonfat varieties, you're getting more saturated fat than you bargained for. Switch to skim milk gradually and your taste buds may never know the difference.

Eggs. If you're on the Step I diet, you can eat up to four egg yolks a week. The Step II diet recommends no more than two egg yolks a week. Remember, it's the saturated fat in the yolk, not the cholesterol, that really does the damage.

Fats and oils. Safflower, corn, sunflower, and soybean oils are polyunsaturated. Olive and canola oils are monounsaturated. Both types will help lower your cholesterol, but only if you use them in small amounts.

Buy soft, tub margarine instead of the hard, stick versions, which are high in trans fatty acids. Stay away from animal products like butter and lard and vegetable fats like coconut oil, palm oil, and hydrogenated shortenings. They are loaded with saturated fat.

Some of these choices may be difficult for you, but it might help to realize that even the smallest changes can make a difference. For every percent of saturated fat calories you stop eating, your bad cholesterol level also drops about 1 percent. It doesn't take long for that to add up.

Fruits and vegetables. Indulge yourself. These super foods are a great source of fiber, vitamins, and minerals and are low in calories, sodium, and fat. There are only a few you should stay away from — coconut, avocados, and olives — because they are high in fat.

Grains and legumes. Peas, beans, and whole-grain foods are not only rich sources of fiber, they lower cholesterol as well.

For more information on any of these plans, visit your local library or bookstore. You'll be able to find more recipes or lengthier explanations about some of the lifestyle changes involved.

Eggs and Egg Substitutes

How to unscramble the cholesterol confusion

Eggs are a quick meal and a basic ingredient in almost everything you slip into the oven. They are essential for summer picnics, traditional holiday fare, and Grandma's light-as-a-feather cake recipe. And because eggs are rich in protein, vitamins, iron, and minerals, they can be a valuable addition to a healthy diet.

But egg yolks have taken a beating lately because they contain cholesterol. The American Heart Association recommends that most people limit their intake of cholesterol to 300 milligrams (mg) per day. The average large egg contains about 213 to 220 mg of cholesterol. That's most of your day's allowance right there. However, this doesn't have to mean the end of French toast and omelets — as long as you understand the bigger picture.

In the fight against cholesterol, saturated fat is your biggest enemy because your body uses it to make cholesterol. The best way to control your cholesterol level is to eat less saturated fat.

Egg yolks contain saturated fat. Not a lot, less than 2 grams, but you should take it into consideration when planning your diet. Just for comparison, 1 ounce of American cheese contains over 5 grams of saturated fat. One 3 1/2-ounce serving of sirloin contains over 9 grams. A glass of skim milk, on the other hand, has less than half a gram.

Naturally, the less saturated fat you eat, the lower your risk of developing heart disease. To keep your cholesterol at a healthy level, experts recommend less than 10 percent of your day's calories should come from saturated fat. So, if you want to enjoy eggs occasionally, eat fewer high-cholesterol, high-fat foods at your other meals. Go ahead and indulge in that three-egg omelet for Sunday brunch as long as you cut back on meat and whole dairy products the rest of the week. In fact, the American Heart Association says about four egg yolks a week is all right for people with normal cholesterol. The tricky part is counting the hidden eggs in your food. One serving of a baked good counts as one-half an egg yolk.

Instead of frying your eggs in butter, try poaching or using a nonfat vegetable spray to cut down on fat — and hold the cheese and the side of bacon with that omelet. To make an all-round healthier meal, serve your eggs with vegetables, fruits, whole-grain breads, and low-fat cheese.

Perhaps the most convincing argument in favor of eggs comes from a study conducted at the Northwest Lipid Research Center in Seattle. Over 100 people, around 50 years old and with high cholesterol, were put on a low-fat diet. Half of the people were fed two eggs a day, while the other half got an egg substitute. Not everyone in the egg group increased their cholesterol levels — only those who already had high amounts of triglycerides, a type of fat, in their bloodstreams.

	Total fat in grams	Saturated fat in grams	Cholesterol in milligrams	Protein in grams	Vitamin A in IU	Folate in micrograms	Vitamin B12 in micrograms
Recommended amount for women over 50	67*	22*	Less than 300	46	2300	400	2.4
Recommended amount for men over 50	67*	22*	Less than 300	56	3000	400	2.4
Whole egg	5.01	1.55	213	6.25	317	23	.50
Egg yolk	5.12	1.59	213	2.78	323	24	.52
Egg white	0	0	0	3.52	0	1	.07
Liquid substitute (3 tablespoons)	1.56	.31	.47	5.64	169.2	7.05	.01
Powder substitute (2 teaspoons)	1.29	.37	56.63	5.50	121.8	12.38	.35

*based on a 2,000-calorie-a-day diet

No yolk — egg whites are 'eggcellent' for your heart

You've whipped them into meringue, you've brushed them on homemade bread, and maybe you've even used them as a facial, but egg whites are also an important weapon in the battle against high cholesterol.

Albumen or egg white is high in protein, riboflavin, and lysine, and it does almost everything whole eggs do. All without one smidgen of fat or cholesterol.

A Japanese study compared cholesterol levels in three different groups of people. One group got about 30 percent of its total protein from egg whites, one from tofu, and the last from cheese. The egg white group lowered its total cholesterol levels as much as the tofu group and more than the cheese group. In addition, it raised its good HDL cholesterol levels more than either the cheese or tofu group.

If you like the idea of cutting down on the yolks, but all that cracking and separating is not for you, look for dried egg whites in stores that sell cake decorating supplies. "Just Whites" is one brand. Simply add water and use in your favorite recipe.

🐾 🐾 🐾

Vitamin D — the 'sunshine' vitamin — from eggs

Egg yolks are one of the few natural food sources of vitamin D, containing about 0.65 micrograms (mcg) per egg. The recommended dietary allowance (RDA) for vitamin D is 10 mcg for 50- to 70-year-olds.

🐾 🐾

Egg stand-ins help clobber cholesterol

Most egg substitutes are made from egg whites, a small amount of vegetable oil, and flavorings. You can buy the powdered variety or the ready-to-use liquid kind at your grocery store. Remember, these substitutes usually have no fat. Without fat, your baked goods could turn out a bit rubbery. You can add an extra tablespoon of oil for a better texture, but don't forget this adds fat and calories.

To make your own egg substitute at home, try this recipe from the Illinois Cooperative Extension Service:

1 tablespoon nonfat dry milk powder
2 egg whites, from large eggs
4 drops yellow food color
1 teaspoon vegetable oil

Mix the first two ingredients, then blend in the food color and oil. This yields about 1/4 cup, or the equivalent of one large egg. Not only does this egg substitute have a bit more protein, it's much lower in cholesterol — about 200 mg less.

Here are several other ways to replace an egg in your favorite recipe:

- blend 2 ounces of soft tofu with water

- mash one-half a banana

- use 1/4 cup applesauce or pureed fruit

- blend 1 tablespoon flaxseed with 3 tablespoons water

- use 1 teaspoon soy flour and 1 tablespoon water

- mix 1 teaspoon cornstarch with 2 tablespoons water

Crack down on egg boredom

Tired of the same old omelet? Fill it with something tasty and nutritious. Here are a few ideas, courtesy of the California Egg Commission, that are sure to put some zip in your eggs, whether you need dinner in a hurry or an out-of-the-ordinary brunch.

- 1 cup mashed potatoes. Mix in onion and seasonings, and top omelet with light sour cream or low-fat cheese.

- 3/4 cup fresh fruit. Top with low-fat yogurt or sherbet, garnish with mint and a touch of powdered sugar.

- 1 cup fresh or leftover salad. Sprinkle croutons and low-fat cheese on top. Drizzle with low-fat dressing.

- 1 cup broken tortilla chips. Microwave with low-fat cheese before filling, then garnish with salsa.

- slices of lean deli meats, low-fat cheeses, and any fresh veggies in your fridge.

And what about an egg white omelet? You don't need all those whole eggs to get the flavor and texture you love. Simply separate out all but one yolk and scramble as normal. For more body, add one tablespoon of low-fat cottage cheese for every yolk you leave out.

Designer eggs land on the sunny side of nutrition

It was just a matter of time before someone built a better egg. Universities and corporations have spent a lot of time and money trying to improve upon Mother Nature. What they've come up with are not just better eggs, but a glimpse into the future of food technology.

There are several designer eggs on the market. Here are some of the brands you might find in your dairy case:

Omega 3 Eggs (Egg Innovations). Developed and patented at the University of Wisconsin, each one of these specially formulated eggs contains 150 mg of omega-3 fatty acids. In addition, you get 17 percent less cholesterol and 300 percent more vitamin E than in a natural egg.

EggsPlus (Pilgrims Pride). Although these designer eggs have the same amount of fat and cholesterol as regular eggs, they have 200 mg of omega 3 fatty acids, 1,100 mg of omega 6 fatty acids, and six times the vitamin E of an average egg.

Are these new and improved eggs really all they're cracked up to be?

When you go shopping, the first thing you'll notice is the price. These designer eggs aren't cheap. They range from $2 per dozen up to $7. Only you can decide if the price is worth the possible health benefits.

You may have heard rumblings of false advertising on some products. You can stay informed on issues like this through FDA and Federal Trade Commission press releases.

Remember, designer eggs are still in their infancy. As the industry learns and grows, processes and marketing will improve. You could be sitting down to the breakfast of the future.

🐌 🐌 🐌

Using your head

Wonder what to do with all those extra egg yolks now that you're eating more heart-healthy? Use them as a hair conditioner. They won't affect your cholesterol one bit.

🐌 🐌

Crustless Seafood Quiche

4 eggs
1 cup light sour cream
1 cup low-fat cottage cheese
1/2 cup Parmesan cheese
4 tablespoons flour
1 teaspoon onion powder
1/4 teaspoon salt
1 can (4 ounces) mushrooms, drained
2 cups (1/2 pound) shredded Monterey Jack cheese

In a blender combine first 7 ingredients. Blend until smooth.

Arrange mushrooms, cheese, and seafood filling in quiche dish. Pour blended ingredients over.

Bake at 350 degrees F. for 45 minutes or until knife inserted in center comes out clean. Let stand 5 minutes before cutting.

For variety: Make one half quiche filled with shrimp and other side salmon, then pour blended mixture over all. Excellent cold.

Filling #1:
8 ounces salad shrimp
1 teaspoon lemon rind
1 tablespoon chopped green onion tops

Filling #2:
8 ounces crab
1 teaspoon lemon rind
1/4 cup sliced almonds

Filling #3:
1 can (15 1/2 ounces) red salmon, flaked
1/2 teaspoon dill weed
1 cup grated cheddar cheese (instead of one of the cups of Jack cheese)

Makes 8 servings

Per serving: 215 Calories; 12g Fat (7g from saturated fat) (51% calories from fat); 20g Protein; 6g Carbohydrate; 174mg Cholesterol; 495mg Sodium

Reprinted with permission from The Alaska Seafood Cookbook
www.state.ak.us/local/akpages/COMMERCE/asmihp.htm

Red and Yellow Pepper Omelets

1 teaspoon olive oil
4 egg whites
1/2 teaspoon dried basil
2 teaspoons grated Parmesan cheese, divided
1 sweet red pepper, thinly sliced
1 yellow pepper, thinly sliced
1/4 teaspoon black pepper

In a large non-stick frying pan over medium heat, warm oil; add the red peppers and yellow peppers; cook stirring frequently for 4 to 5 minutes. Keep warm over low heat. In a small bowl, lightly whisk together the egg whites, basil and black pepper. Coat a small non-stick frying pan with non-stick spray. Warm over medium-high heat for 1 minute. Add half of the egg mixture, swirling the pan to evenly coat the bottom. Cook for 30 seconds or until the eggs are set. Carefully loosen and flip; cook for 1 minute, or until firm. Sprinkle half of the peppers over the eggs. Fold to enclose the filling. Transfer to a plate. Sprinkle with 1 teaspoon of the Parmesan. Repeat with the remaining egg mixture, peppers and 1 teaspoon Parmesan.

Makes 2 servings.

Nutritional Analysis Per Serving: Calories, 85; Fat, 3g; Fiber, 1.2g; Cholesterol, 2mg; Sodium, 151mg; percent calories from fat, 32%.

Spanish Omelet

2 baked potatoes, diced
2 cups fat-free egg substitute
1 large tomato, seeded and diced
2 tablespoons minced fresh parsley
2 cloves garlic, minced
1 teaspoon olive oil
1 large onion, minced
2 teaspoons margarine

In a large non-stick frying pan over medium heat, cook the potatoes, onions, tomatoes, parsley and garlic in the oil until most of liquid has evaporated from the tomatoes. Transfer to a large bowl and stir in eggs. Wipe out the frying pan then place it over medium-high heat and let stand for about 2 minutes. Add 1 teaspoon margarine and swirl the pan to distribute. Add half of the egg mixture; lift and rotate pan so that the eggs are evenly distributed. As the eggs set around the edges, lift them to allow uncooked portions to flow underneath. Turn the heat to low, cover the pan and cook until the top is set. Invert onto a serving plate. Cut into wedges. Repeat with the remaining 1 teaspoon margarine and egg mixture.

Makes 4 servings.

Nutritional Analysis Per Serving: Calories, 211; Fat, 3.3g; Fiber, 3.6g; Cholesterol, 0mg; Sodium, 174mg; percent calories from fat, 14%.

Estrogen

Be cautious of hormone therapy

Researchers recently stopped a large hormone replacement therapy (HRT) study because they were concerned about health risks. Five years into the study, they were startled to see a significant increase in heart disease risk as well as invasive breast cancer. Their research showed:

- a 26 percent rise in breast cancer
- 22 percent more cardiovascular disease
- a 29 percent increase in heart attacks
- a 41 percent jump in stroke
- twice the rate of blood clots

That translates into seven to eight more cancer or heart disease cases per 10,000 HRT users each year. That may not seem like a lot, but when you look at the population as a whole, it could mean thousands more health problems over time.

Estrogen also slightly raises your risk of blood clots in your veins, often in your legs, that can clog up a vessel and stop the blood supply to a vital organ. One study says estrogen may increase your risk of asthma. Other possible side effects of HRT are bleeding, bloating, cramps, and breast tenderness.

As a result, the Food and Drug Administration (FDA) now advises doctors to prescribe HRT only when benefits clearly outweigh health risks, just long enough for successful treatment, and at the lowest effective dose. What's more, women should consider non-HRT treatments for vaginal dryness and osteoporosis. If your risk for breast cancer is high, HRT may not be a good option for you.

Reversing the long-held notion that HRT protects against heart disease, both the FDA and American Heart Association now warn against using hormone therapy to reduce the chances of heart problems.

Heart disease risk factors

- Age 55 or older
- 20 to 30 percent overweight
- Excess weight around waist (apple-shaped)
- Family history (especially a parent who had a heart attack at an early age)
- A high-stress lifestyle
- Cigarette smoking
- High blood cholesterol
- High blood pressure
- Diabetes
- Physical inactivity

Breast cancer risk factors

- Strong family history (mother or sister with breast cancer)
- High-fat diet
- High-alcohol intake

- Early puberty (before 13)
- Late menopause (after 50)
- Not having breast-fed any children

🐌 🐌 🐌

Check out the future of hormone therapy

What if you could get all the heart-saving advantages of estrogen without the risks?

Scientists are working on new drugs that offer the good effects of estrogen on your bones, without the bad effects on your uterus, heart, and breasts. These 'smart estrogens' or SERMs (selective estrogen receptor modulators) take the worry out of hormone therapy while still offering many of the heart-healthy benefits.

🐌 🐌

A natural way to boost your estrogen

Did you know plants have hormones, too? Called phyto-estrogens, these natural chemicals are weaker versions of human estrogen. When you eat foods containing phytoestro-gens, they are broken down in your body and do many of the same things your own estrogen does.

Researchers first became interested in these plant estrogens when they discovered that Asian people, who eat large amounts of soy and other estrogen-containing plants, have fewer cases of breast cancer and heart disease. They also found that women in these countries suffered from fewer of the common Western menopause symptoms. For more information on these studies, see *The Asian diet* in the *Eating plans* chapter.

As part of an ordinary diet, phytoestrogens are safe and can even be heart-healthy. But doctors don't recommend supplementing with large amounts of phytoestrogen pills since there can be serious side effects. And they don't believe diet alone can get your hormones back in balance.

If you want to boost your estrogen naturally, try adding these phytoestrogens to your diet — garlic, parsley, dates, cherries, apples, carrots, potatoes, beans, wheat, rice, flaxseed, and even coffee. But perhaps the most well-known food source of phytoestrogens is the soybean. You can read more about soy and soy foods in the *Soy* chapter.

Exercise

6 reasons to get your body moving

Experts say a lack of exercise is as much a heart disease risk factor as high cholesterol, cigarette smoking, and high blood pressure. Here's how exercising can help you shape up to a healthier heart.

Peels off pounds. Carrying around excess weight is a sure route to high cholesterol, high blood pressure, and diabetes. If you want to lose weight, you must burn up more calories than you take in, and exercise can help. The best results come from combining aerobic exercise, like brisk walking or jogging, with a low-fat diet.

Keeps arteries flexible. As you age, your blood vessels become less flexible. When your muscles signal a need for more oxygen and nutrients, your arteries can't dilate to allow more blood to flow through. Your heart has to work harder, which increases your heart rate and blood pressure. By exercising regularly, you are actually keeping your arteries in shape, not just your muscles.

Improves cholesterol levels. There's no doubt about it — regular exercise lowers total and bad LDL cholesterol and increases good HDL cholesterol. Some studies have found that exercise can improve cholesterol levels as much as medication, without the side effects.

Lowers heart attack risk. Do you worry that exercising will bring on a heart attack? If you never work out and suddenly do something strenuous, there is some risk. The good news is regular exercise will lower this risk. If your heart is used to moderate exercise, say four or five workouts a week, then some heavy exertion shouldn't be dangerous. Pass that snow shovel on to someone else, though, if you don't exercise regularly.

Speeds recovery time. If you have suffered a heart attack or other heart-related injury, here's good motivation to start some kind of exercise program. Studies have shown that if you become active right away, you are more likely to be discharged earlier from the hospital and return to your usual activities.

Lifts your spirits. When you do something physical, you just plain feel better. Although depression is common after a heart attack, it will usually go away on its own. In the meantime, exercise will help to lessen that gloomy feeling. You'll feel an emotional lift knowing you are doing something good for your body. You'll also feel a very real physical charge when your body releases chemicals called endorphins. These block pain and give you a sense of well-being.

How to choose the workout that's right for you

Most people were thrilled to hear reports that a small amount of frequent exercise did their hearts good. This is the "little bit goes a long way" theory. Researchers examined over 200 postmenopausal women who suffered from heart disease and found that 30 to 45 minutes of walking, three times a week, was enough to decrease their risk of heart attack by 50 percent.

Do you do things whole-heartedly? Then you'll like the research that defends the "more is better" theory. Some studies have proven that long-distance runners reduce their blood pressure and their need for blood pressure medication more than those who run shorter distances. In addition, their risk of heart disease is 30 percent lower.

According to another study, if you are beginning an exercise program, you must run eight to 10 miles per week in order to make any noticeable changes in your levels of HDL cholesterol. That's more action than most people can handle.

And last, there are those who say you need intense workouts that really get your heart going if you want to see any health benefits.

If all this is just too confusing, base your exercise program on what the American Heart Association recommends — minimize risk and maximize benefit. This means choosing a program that will bring you the most improvement without jeopardizing your health.

If you decide on low-intensity exercises, such as walking or biking, you'll see healthy results, but it will take longer. The advantages of these exercises are less stress on your body and less risk of injury. If you choose something more strenuous, like jogging, you will see faster results, but you're also more likely to have bone or joint injuries.

🐞 🐞 🐞

What to do before you get started

If you're over 40, moderate walking is considered safe, but if you want to do something more vigorous, you'll need a physical exam and an exercise test. This test will evaluate how your body reacts to exercise. Based on your test results, your doctor can help you decide what kind of exercise is best for you.

Although exercise testing is considered safe, the American Heart Association says if you suffer from angina, uncontrolled congestive heart failure, or arrhythmia, this test could be dangerous for you.

🐞 🐞

Measuring how hard you're working

Moderate exercise means you are maintaining your heart rate at 40 to 60 percent of your maximum heart rate. Exercise intensities greater than 60 percent are called vigorous or intense.

To maximize your aerobic benefits from exercising, you need to determine your maximum heart rate and your target heart rate (the number of heartbeats per minute you want to achieve during exercise). For maximum benefits, you should maintain your target heart rate for at least 20 minutes.

To find your maximum heart rate:

1. Start with the number 220   **220**
2. Subtract your age (50, for example)   **-   50**
3. The answer is your maximum heart rate   **170**

To find your target heart rate at 60 percent intensity:

1. Take your maximum heart rate   **170**
2. Multiply your maximum heart rate by 0.6   x   **0.6**
3. The answer is your target heart rate   **102**

If you want to exercise at 80 percent intensity, multiply your maximum heart rate by 0.8.

If you want to know how hard your heart is working or if you are near your target heart rate, find your pulse and count the number of heartbeats in 10 seconds. Multiply this number by six to get the number of times your heart is beating in one minute. Compare your target heart rate to your pulse rate to see if you're working at the right intensity.

According to some experts, your body can only burn fat when you exercise aerobically, which increases the amount of oxygen your body needs. For the greatest benefits, your aerobic exercise should raise your heart rate from 60 to 80 percent of its maximum rate.

After exercising at this level for 20 minutes, your body will begin to consume fat for fuel. On the other hand, if your workout pushes your heart rate above 85 percent of the maximum level, this is considered anaerobic or "without air" exercise. At this point, your body automatically switches over to the higher test fuels, carbohydrates and protein, leaving the fat right where you don't want it.

8 things to remember about exercising

You'll find as many exercise programs as there are fitness experts. Although each will promise heart benefits and healthy results, you'll find it helpful to follow these general guidelines:

Do it often. To make a lasting difference, exercise every other day. Your body needs activity on a regular basis. Sometimes it's hard to hang in there, but don't quit. Exercising for just a few weeks won't make any difference to your cholesterol levels.

Warm it up. Warming up can decrease stress on your heart. If you jump right into a strenuous exercise, your heart will probably not get enough blood flow and oxygen right away. Warming up slowly increases blood flow to the heart, which could reduce your risk of a heart attack.

Many people think stretching before exercise is a good way to warm up, but stretching cold muscles could actually cause an injury. The best way to warm up is to gradually begin whatever activity you plan to be doing. If you run, begin by walking. If you swim, begin with leisurely laps, slowly getting faster. This gradual increase warms up the specific muscles you will be using during exercise. You'll need to warm up more in cold weather and less in hot weather. If you plan to exercise outdoors in cold weather, try warming up inside so you won't have to remove extra clothing as you get warmer.

Cool it down. Cooling down is just as important as warming up because it helps to remove some chemical by-products of exercise from your muscles. It also helps lower levels of adrenaline in your bloodstream, which increase during exercise. If this extra adrenaline remains in your bloodstream during rest, it can place extra stress on your heart. Sudden inactivity after vigorous exercise can even cause blood to pool, especially in your legs. This could lead to lightheadedness and decreased blood flow to your heart. In cold weather, cool down indoors to help prevent chills by slowing the loss of body heat.

Stretch it out. Bring down the pace of your workout slowly, and then stretch those muscles. This will help prevent some of the stiffness you may experience after exercise.

Take time to digest. Wait at least two hours after a meal before you exercise. That gives your digestive system time to move everything through your intestines. Otherwise, you might get cramps, feel nauseated, or faint.

Know your limits. Set reasonable and safe goals that won't cause more problems than benefits. If it's hot, slow it down and drink lots of water. If you've got a cold, the flu, or a fever, take a few days off from your routine. Your body needs to concentrate on recovering.

Make it fun. Exercise shouldn't feel like work. Give your body time to adjust to a new routine, then gradually make it harder. You are much more likely to stick with a program you enjoy, so be creative. And if you find a buddy to exercise with, you'll both be more motivated.

Watch out for warning signs. You may experience certain symptoms, even during the mildest forms of exercise. Some are normal. Others are warning signs that you need immediate medical attention. Talk to your doctor about these and other indications of possible trouble:

- back or joint pain
- faintness or light-headedness during exercise or nausea afterward
- shortness of breath
- an aching, burning, or tightness in your upper body
- extreme fatigue or sleeplessness

Walk your way to a healthy heart

Why is walking the first type of exercise your doctor recommends? It's cheap; the risk of injury is extremely low; it requires no special equipment, except for a good pair of walking shoes; and it can be just as beneficial as more intense exercise.

Walking helps lower your blood pressure, raise your HDL cholesterol, burn body fat, and increase your fitness level. It gets you started and, hopefully, hooked on an exercise program, and it can pave the way for something more intense later on.

Walking is usually the first and only exercise your doctor will recommend after a heart attack. You'll begin at a slow, regular pace, for no more than 10 minutes, and gradually work your way up to longer sessions.

Find a route where the path is smooth and traffic is light. Lighting and visibility are also important for your safety. Shopping malls are great places to walk, since you can continue this very healthy activity in any kind of weather.

Choose different exercises for different needs

Aerobic exercise. Also called endurance exercises, these include any activities that increase the amount of oxygen you need to fuel your muscles. Brisk walking, running, cycling, dancing, rowing, swimming, and skating are just a few examples. Aerobic exercise increases your heart rate and stamina and may reduce blood pressure. It also prevents the build up of fatty deposits in your arteries and helps prevent blood clots.

Anaerobic exercise. This type of exercise focuses on specific muscles for short but intense periods of time. Weight lifting, baseball, and golf (riding in a cart) are anaerobic exercises. Also called muscle training, anaerobic exercises can be unhealthy if you do them for too long at one time. Your body can begin to burn its store of carbohydrates and protein for fuel instead of burning fats.

Calisthenics. These are the gymnastic-type exercises you did in gym class, like push-ups and sit-ups. They increase your heart rate and build strength.

Cardiovascular exercises. These exercises use large muscle groups, like those in your arms and legs. Usually you do these kinds of exercises continuously, in a certain rhythm. Most cardiovascular exercises are also aerobic. They increase your heart rate, lower blood pressure, enlarge arteries, and improve the oxygen supply to your muscles.

Flexibility activities. Slow, concentrated movements that involve stretching, relaxing, and breathing deeply, like tai chi and yoga, increase flexibility. They also lower blood pressure, increase the range of motion of your joints, and improve balance. See the *Movement therapy* chapter for more information on activities like these.

Isometric exercises. Isometrics involve tightening muscles without actually moving any joints. An example is simply pressing your palms together. These fall under the category of anaerobic exercises, since you don't use up a lot of oxygen doing them. They can strengthen your muscles and keep your joints stable.

Isotonic exercises. When you contract muscles and move a joint at the same time, you are doing an isotonic exercise. Leg lifts are an example of isotonic exercise. This type of exercise can strengthen your muscles.

Resistance training. This kind of exercising is also called strength or weight training. It's a combination of isometric and isotonic exercises — muscle tightening with small movements. Lifting free weights is a type of resistance training. It can cause a temporary rise in your blood pressure if you don't breathe properly while you are doing them. Also, people with heart conditions should be careful to avoid lifting extremely heavy weights. You can improve your condition just as much by doing more repetitions with moderate weights. Resistance training can help lower cholesterol; increase your strength and flexibility; and strengthen muscles, tendons, and ligaments.

High blood pressure? Exercise common sense

If you have high blood pressure, you may have been advised to avoid exercise since you could be at a higher risk of suffering a heart attack. Concern about exercise-induced heart attacks has led many doctors to tell their patients to toss their tennis shoes.

Though strenuous exercise can cause a temporary increase in blood pressure, regular exercise will eventually lower blood pressure. And statistics show that if you are inactive you have up to a 50 percent greater risk of developing high blood pressure. Exercise helps you lose weight, and weight loss contributes to lower blood pressure.

If you have severe high blood pressure, follow your doctor's advice to get it under control. Once it's under control, ask your doctor if you can begin aerobic activities, such as jogging or brisk walking. Three to five sessions per week for 20 to 60 minutes should soon produce results.

People who have high blood pressure should avoid weight training because lifting heavy weights can cause a sharp rise in blood pressure. However, circuit training, which uses lighter weights with more repetitions, may be a good alternative. The most effective circuit training program consists of 10 to 15 repetitions in 30 to 45 seconds with a 30 to 50 percent resistance load. The resistance load is a percentage of the maximum weight you can lift in a single repetition. You should rest 15 to 30 seconds between exercises and perform about 10 to 12 exercises two or three times per session.

Caffeine and exercise may not mix well for those with high blood pressure. Be aware that caffeine can temporarily cause a sharp increase in blood pressure, just as exercise can. Mixing the two at the same time may be asking for trouble.

Don't let high blood pressure keep you from the gym or the tennis courts. Just exercise a little common sense, and enjoy the benefits exercise can bring.

Head pain sometimes spells heart trouble

If your headaches begin during exercise, then go away when you rest, it may be a sign of heart disease.

Researchers recently found this to be the case with seven patients who did not suffer any signs of heart problems but had other risk factors, such as high blood pressure, a history of smoking, or heart disease in the family.

Researchers at the Headache Unit at Montefiore Medical Center in New York have several theories of how an otherwise silent heart condition can cause severe headaches. They believe it's possible that referred chest pain travels along nerves from the heart to the head where it's more noticeable. Or, the diseased heart causes more pressure in the head because of poor circulation.

It's not the headache that is a cause of concern, but the fact that these people had no other symptoms of heart disease. Although these so-called cardiac headaches are rare, they could be your body's way of alerting you to more serious trouble. So if you end your workouts with a throbbing head, have your doctor check your heart.

Fat Substitutes

The latest trend — indulging without guilt

What if all your favorite high-fat foods suddenly contained zero grams of fat but tasted exactly the same? It may sound too good to be true, but it's now possible with the use of fat substitutes or replacers, ingredients that take the place of fat in foods and drinks.

Fat substitutes are most often made from common food ingredients, but they can also be man-made. They give your favorite foods the taste and texture of fat without adding any fat, calories, or cholesterol.

Since different foods require different kinds of fat, the industry came up with different kinds of fat substitutes. Some work well in fried foods, while others break down in heat and are better suited for frozen foods. Sometimes, more than one kind of substitute is used in a single food in order to keep the original flavors.

When real fat is removed from a product, much of the flavor goes with it. That's why manufacturers of some low-fat foods add extra salt or sugar. If you have high blood pressure, make sure you read labels for sodium content.

Even though a fat substitute lowers the calorie and fat content of a food, it does not make it more nutritious. That fat-free chocolate cake will still have the same amount of vitamins, minerals, protein, fiber, and sugar as before. Many people have been known to actually gain weight on low-fat diets because they think fat-free means calorie-free.

The debate on the safety and role of fat substitutes in a healthy diet will most likely continue until more information on the long-term effects is available.

Everything you need to know about fat substitutes

New ingredients and processes are continually being investigated by food technologists to help them come up with better fat substitutes. There are three main types of fat substitutes — carbohydrate-based, protein-based, and fat-based.

Carbohydrate-based. These are the most common type. They are natural plant ingredients like cellulose, maltodextrins, gums, starches, fiber, and polydextrose. These soak up water and create a slippery, fat-like feel to foods. You've probably seen ingredients like modified food starch or guar gum on labels for reduced-fat and fat-free foods. They've been used for years to thicken certain products and to increase the shelf life of processed foods. These fat substitutes contain calories, but fewer than regular fat.

Z-Trim is a carbohydrate-based fat substitute developed by the U.S. Department of Agriculture. It's a powder made from the outer husk, or bran, of various grains such as soybeans, corn, wheat, rice, or oats. When the powder absorbs water, it swells and gives food the same smooth "mouth feel" as fat. In addition to being a great fat substitute, Z-Trim adds lots of natural fiber without any calories. It has been used in hamburger, deli meats, and cheeses.

Another carbohydrate-based fat substitute is Oatrim. Made from oat starch and oat fiber, it's combined into a gel that replaces butter or oil in many foods. Because of its high fiber content, Oatrim can help to lower cholesterol as it reduces the amount of fat. It has no flavor, so you won't be able to taste any difference in your food. It has even been used to replace half of the whipping cream in candy with good results.

Other brand names of carbohydrate-based fat substitutes include: Avicel, Methocel, Solka-Floc, Amylum, N-Oil, Opta, Oat Fiber, Snowite, Ultracel, Kelcogel, Keltrol, Slendid, Fruitafit, Fibruline, CrystaLean, Lorelite, Lycadex, Maltrin, Beta-Trim, TrimChoice, Litesse, Sta-Lite, and Sta-Slim.

Protein-based. These have only been around for about 10 years. They are made by shaping protein, usually egg whites or dairy protein, into tiny round particles. These microscopic balls roll around easily in your mouth, making you think you're eating a smooth and creamy fat. You cannot fry with protein-based substitutes, but they are used in products like cheese, margarine, salad dressing, soup, ice cream, and bread. If you are on a protein-restricted diet, talk to your doctor before eating protein-based fat substitutes.

Simplesse is a well-known protein-based fat substitute. It can either be made from egg whites and used in frozen desserts, or from milk protein and used in cooked foods. It is all natural, low in calories, and has zero cholesterol. You may have seen it in fat-free versions of mayonnaise, yogurt, cheese spreads, salad dressings, and ice cream.

Dairy-Lo, K-Blazer, Ultra-Bake, Ultra-Freeze, and Lita are also brand names of protein-based fat substitutes.

Fat-based. These taste more like fat than the other substitutes because they really contain fat. They are simply fat molecules that have had their chemical structure changed so your body can't digest them.

These chemical fat substitutes must be approved by the Food and Drug Administration (FDA) since they aren't naturally occurring ingredients. The food industry is very excited about fat-based substitutes since they can be used in baking or frying. Chips, pretzels, popcorn, and other high-fat snack foods are the first products to be tested with new fat-based substitutes.

Olestra, a combination of sugar and fatty acids from vegetable oil, is currently the biggest news in fat substitutes. The flurry of excitement in the media and the food industry is because calorie-free olestra, also known as Olean, is the first fat replacer that can be used under high heat conditions, like frying.

Although it has received FDA approval and is already in several snack products, this fat substitute remains under a heavy cloud of controversy.

How it works is really quite simple. The olestra molecule is too large to pass through the walls of your intestines and on into your bloodstream. It just slides down your digestive system and keeps on going. Your mouth gets the taste and feel of a high-fat food, but your body never actually absorbs any fat.

One of the problems with olestra is that it acts like a laxative on some people, causing cramping and diarrhea. It also carries important nutrients with it on its way out. Vitamins A, D, E, and K, and carotenoids like beta carotene and lycopene are usually lost.

Supporters of olestra say the stomach problems only occur in people who have a sensitivity to undigested fat. Other researchers found that some people have similar reactions when they make any change to their regular diet, like eating more fiber, for instance.

Whatever the reason, the FDA hopes to avoid problems by requiring products containing olestra to be fortified with vitamins A, D, E, and K to make up for the amount lost. Also, food manufacturers using olestra must print this warning on their products: "Olestra may cause abdominal cramping and loose stools. Olestra inhibits the absorption of some vitamins and other nutrients. Vitamins A, D, E, and K have been added." And Procter & Gamble, the manufacturer of olestra, has been required to study the long-term effects of this fat substitute on humans.

Olestra isn't the only fat-based substitute being used. The others include Benefat, Dur-Lo, EC, and Caprenin.

Enjoy natural fat substitutes from your kitchen

Instead of	calories	fat (g)	Use	calories	fat (g)
1 cup buttered bread crumbs	392	5	1 cup crushed corn flakes	110	0
2 tablespoons margarine for baking	201	23	2 tablespoons light corn syrup for baking	113	0
1 cup sour cream	493	48	1 cup low-fat yogurt	144	0
1 egg	79	6	2 egg whites	32	0
1 tablespoon mayonnaise	102	11	1 tablespoon mustard	10	1
1/2 cup heavy cream for thickening	410	44	1/2 cup pureed potato for thickening	67	0
1/2 cup vegetable oil in salad dressings	964	109	1/2 cup rice puree* in salad dressings	120	0
1/2 cup vegetable oil for baking	964	109	1/2 cup applesauce for baking	97	0
1 tablespoon oil for stir-fry	120	14	1 tablespoon fat-free chicken broth for stir-fry	2	0
1 cup nondairy whipped topping	224	4	1 cup evaporated skim milk, partially frozen whipped	215	1
1 tablespoon solid shortening	100	11	3 seconds of nonstick cooking spray	6	1

Instead of	calories	fat (g)	Use	calories	fat (g)
1 ounce cream cheese	100	10	1 ounce low-fat ricotta	32	2
1 tablespoon oil for baking	120	14	4 ounces soft tofu for baking	50	2
1 cup whole milk for baking	156	9	1 cup low-fat buttermilk for baking	99	2
3 slices (19 grams) bacon	109	9	1 slice (23 grams) Canadian bacon	43	2
2 tablespoons margarine for baking	201	23	2 tablespoons fat-free cream cheese for baking	25	0
1 patty (85 grams) hamburger	240	17	1 patty (82 grams) ground turkey	193	11
1 square baking chocolate	185	16	3 tablespoons cocoa	122	12

*1/2 cup rice cooked in 4 cups water until very soft then pureed in blender or food processor

Cut the fat with nutrient-packed prunes

The funny-looking prune is enjoying a comeback. You'll find them in trendy entrees and festive salads. They're virtually fat-free, low in calories, and a great source of vitamin A, iron, and potassium. And if you're looking for a heart-healthy snack, it's hard to beat a prune. Packed with fiber — six prunes have over 4 grams — this sweet, year-round fruit can help lower your cholesterol.

One way to get the most heart-healthy benefit out of prunes is to bake with them. Prune puree, also known as dried plum puree, can take the place of butter or oil in your favorite recipe or packaged mix without adding any fat. A general rule is to use half the amount of butter or oil called for in a recipe and replace the rest with half as much prune puree. For example, if a recipe calls for 1 cup of butter, use 1/2 cup butter and replace the second 1/2 cup butter with 1/4 cup prune puree.

Product	Calories	Fat
1 cup prune puree	407	1 gram
1 cup butter	1,600	182 grams
1 cup oil	1,944	218 grams

You can find fruit puree in the cooking oil or baking section of your supermarket, but it's easy to make your own.

Prune puree

8 ounces pitted prunes
6 tablespoons hot water

Combine in food processor or blender and pulse on and off until the prunes are finely chopped and the mixture is the consistency of applesauce. Cover and refrigerate for up to one month. Makes 1 cup.

Fish and Fish Oil

Cast your net for a healthier heart

Ever think a fatty fish could save your life? No, Tubby the Tuna isn't going to rescue you from drowning, but eating fish, like tuna, may be the life preserver that saves you from a heart attack. In fact, if you need to baby your heart, a diet high in fish is better for you than a strictly vegetarian diet. That's because certain seafood contains omega-3 fatty acids, which have been shown to reduce the risk of heart disease. These polyunsaturated fats are found only in cold-water fish, like salmon, sardines, and herring.

What they do is relax the cells lining your blood vessels, which means lower blood pressure and better circulation for you. They also keep your blood from clotting, decreasing your chance of heart attack and stroke. In fact, eating fish several times a week can cut your risk of stroke in half. And omega-3 fatty acids can lower the amount of fats in your blood — fats that can lead to high cholesterol and atherosclerosis.

How much fish do you need to eat? Not as much as you might think. Experts say at least one 3-ounce serving of fatty fish a week, about the size of a cassette tape, is enough to cut your risk of heart disease. But to get more dramatic results, you'd want to visit the fish market up to four times a week. If you really want to see a big drop in your cholesterol, reel in some seafood every day. The Japanese, who have a much lower rate of heart disease than North Americans, eat about one-fourth pound of fish a day.

Fish is a good nutrition decision because it's low in calories, fat, and cholesterol and high in vitamins and minerals. It's also a good source of protein. For a healthy heart, throw back that sirloin and land a tuna steak instead.

If you have avoided fish, especially shrimp, in the past because you thought it was too high in cholesterol, go ahead and pass the cocktail sauce. In a recent study, eating 300 grams of steamed shrimp, containing about 590 milligrams (mg) of cholesterol, every day affected cholesterol levels less than eating two large eggs per day, which contain about 580 mg of cholesterol. Researchers believe the answer to this puzzle is hooked into omega-3.

For your best sources of omega-3, see the following chart. You want to choose the fish with the highest amount of omega-3, but the least amount of fat. In other words, those with the highest percentage of omega-3. You'll find these numbers in the far right column. Portions are based on an uncooked serving size of 100 grams, or approximately 3 to 3 1/2 ounces.

Food	Total fat in grams	Omega-3 in grams	% omega-3 of fat
Atlantic cod	0.7	0.3	43
Alaska King crab	0.8	0.3	38
Striped bass	2.3	0.8	35
Dungeness crab	1.0	0.3	30
European anchovy	4.8	1.4	29
Haddock	0.7	0.2	29
Pink salmon	3.4	1.0	29

Food (continued)	Total fat in grams	Omega-3 in grams	% omega-3 of fat
Shrimp	1.1	0.3	27
Pacific oyster	2.3	0.6	26
Scallops	0.8	0.2	25
Atlantic salmon	5.4	1.2	22
Northern lobster	0.9	0.2	22
Blue mussels	2.2	0.5	22
Sardines in oil	15.5	3.3	21
Flounder	1.0	0.2	20
Tuna	2.5	0.5	20
Atlantic herring	9.0	1.6	18
Mackerel	13.9	2.5	18
Pacific halibut	2.3	0.4	17
Lake trout	9.7	1.6	17
Red snapper	1.2	0.2	17
Rainbow trout	3.4	0.5	15
Pacific herring	13.9	1.7	12
Swordfish	2.1	0.2	10
Sole	1.2	0.1	8
Catfish	4.3	0.3	7

But what if you're not fond of fish? Don't despair. You can actually get omega-3 from certain plants. Of course, oils taken from these plants are some of the most concentrated sources of this good fatty acid. You'll find that rapeseed (canola), walnut, wheat germ, and soybean oils are especially rich in heart-healthy alpha-linolenic acid. But flaxseed oil has probably the highest concentration of omega-3 — over 50 percent. So the next time you're planning a stir-fry, get adventurous with your oil. Your taste buds and your heart will love it.

The following plant foods also contain omega-3; not in large amounts, but enough to make them smart additions to your weekly menu.

Food (100 grams or about 3 1/2 ounces)	Total fat in grams	Omega-3 in grams	% omega-3 of fat
Flaxseed	41.0	2.3	57
Soybeans, sprouted, cooked	4.5	2.1	47
Common dry beans	1.5	0.6	40
Navy beans	0.8	0.3	38
Leeks, raw	2.1	0.7	34
Pinto beans	0.9	0.3	33
Kale, raw	0.7	0.2	29
Spinach, raw	0.4	0.1	25
Strawberries, raw	0.4	0.1	25
English walnuts	61.9	6.8	11
Dry soybeans	21.3	1.6	8
Black walnuts	56.6	3.3	6
Wheat germ	10.9	0.7	6
Oat germ	30.7	1.4	5

In case you're wondering what to fix with all this mouth-watering fish, anything will do, so long as it's low-fat. According to a recent Australian study, you get even more heart-healthy benefits from fish when you combine it with a low-fat diet. Taking off the skin will remove most of the fat and calories, but it won't make any difference in the omega-3 fatty acids. Do your heart a favor and whip up a delicious low-fat fish dish.

☙ ☙ ☙

Chicken — the new catch of the day

Some people have a hard time liking the distinctive flavor of fish. It's just too — well — fishy. If only it tasted more like chicken. But what if you could eat chicken and get all the same omega-3 benefits of fish? Sound like the stuff of science fiction? Perhaps not.

The whole process begins in the ocean with what fish eat — algae. This is where all those good fatty acids come from. Several companies are experimenting with growing their own algae and turning it into feed for chickens. They hope to produce eggs and, eventually, chicken meat that is rich in heart-saving omega-3.

Several designer eggs are already on the market in certain test areas. Read more about them in the *Eggs* chapter. And be on the lookout for heart-healthier chicken, beef, and even pork that may swim into your local meat department in the future.

☙ ☙

Fish + garlic = double trouble for high cholesterol

You know what a clove of garlic can do for the flavor of a nice piece of salmon. And shrimp sautéed in garlic and olive oil is truly a gourmet's delight. Your heart is finally finding out what your taste buds have known all along — fish plus garlic is one winning combination.

Medical researchers have discovered that this one-two punch lowers bad LDL cholesterol more and presents a better ratio of good to bad cholesterol than either food source alone. This is an exciting discovery for people trying to control their cholesterol without taking drugs. A garlic-fish combination may be just what the chef — and the doctor — ordered.

210

High Blood Pressure Lowered Naturally

🐜 🐜 🐜

Cracking the shellfish myth

If lobster is the king of seafood, shrimp is undeniably the prince. But this popular item is still considered by many to be a treat reserved for special occasions only. Lots of people deny themselves shrimp and other tasty shellfish, like oysters, clams, and crab, because they don't believe they're healthy food choices.

If that's the case, you are also denying yourself a delicious meal that's low in fat and calories and high in protein, iron, copper, and zinc. And like other fish, shellfish can be a terrific source of important omega-3 fatty acids.

It is true that shrimp, especially, can be high in cholesterol, but eating it does not seem to raise your cholesterol level. Researchers at Rockefeller University found that a shrimp diet lowered the ratio of total to HDL cholesterol, and of LDL to HDL cholesterol. In other words, by keeping these levels in proportion, the good effects of shrimp cancelled out the bad.

When you're comparing numbers on the following chart, consider that 3-1/2 ounces of roasted white meat chicken, without the skin, has 85 grams of cholesterol. Add to that the fact that shrimp contain almost no fat, and you've got yourself one nutritious, mouthwatering meal.

3-ounce portion (steamed)*	cholesterol (milligrams)	calories	fat (grams)
Scallops	40	90	1
Crab	45	82	1.3
Mussels	48	147	3.8
Clams	57	126	1.7
Lobster	61	83	0.5
Oysters	93	117	4.2
Shrimp	166	84	0.9

*Thoroughly cook all shellfish to avoid food poisoning.

🐜 🐜

Beware of fish oil capsules

Many experts, including the American Heart Association, do not recommend taking fish oil capsules. The benefits of supplementing have not been proven and many people experience side effects like:

- stomach upset
- nosebleeds
- bruising
- weight gain

In addition, some supplements may contain cholesterol, pesticides, or toxic amounts of vitamins A and D. Why spend a lot of money on supplements when you can get a safer, cheaper, and better dose of omega-3 naturally, from your grocery store?

Elegant Baked Snapper

2 pounds snapper fillets
1 cup light sour cream
1 teaspoon seafood seasoning
1 teaspoon dill weed
1/2 to 1/4 cup finely minced onion
1/2 teaspoon pepper
3/4 cup grated cheddar cheese

Place fillets in a baking dish and sprinkle with dill weed.

Mix the light sour cream, seafood seasoning, and pepper together and use a rubber scraper to "frost" the mixture over the fillets.

Sprinkle with the chopped onion and the grated cheddar cheese.

Bake at 400 degrees F. until lightly browned and the fish flakes easily with a fork when tested in the center.

Microwave version:

Prepare as above, cover, and cook in the microwave on high for 8 minutes. Test and continue to cook until the fish flakes easily. Brown in the oven (lightly).

Makes 6 servings

Per serving: 228 Calories; 8g Fat (3g from saturated fat) (31% calories from fat); 36g Protein; 2g Carbohydrate; 74mg Cholesterol; 195mg Sodium

Reprinted with permission from the Alaska Seafood Marketing Institute
www.state.ak.us/local/akpages/COMMERCE/asmihp.htm

Salmon Fettuccine

1 can (7 1/2 ounces) Alaska salmon
2 tablespoons margarine
1/4 cup flour
2 1/2 cups hot low-fat milk
2 tablespoons sherry
2 tablespoons sliced green onions
3/4 teaspoon Dijon mustard
3/4 teaspoon dill weed
black pepper to taste
8 ounces fettuccine noodles
1 tablespoon chopped parsley

Drain and flake salmon. Set aside.

Melt margarine in a medium saucepan over medium heat. Remove from heat and whisk in flour. Cook, stirring constantly, for 2-3 minutes.

Whisk in milk and sherry; cook, stirring frequently, for 15 minutes.

Stir in flaked salmon and remaining ingredients except fettuccine and parsley. Cook 2-3 more minutes, until heated through.

Meanwhile, cook pasta according to package directions; drain and place on serving platter. Spoon sauce over pasta and sprinkle with parsley to serve.

Makes 4 appetizer servings or 2 main dish servings

Per serving: 438 Calories; 12g Fat (3g from saturated fat) (24% calories from fat); 24g Protein; 56g Carbohydrate; 35mg Cholesterol; 456mg Sodium

Reprinted with permission from the Alaska Seafood Marketing Institute. www.state.ak.us/local/akpages/COMMERCE/asmihp.htm

Flaxseed

Harvest the benefits of this wonder plant

You can paint with it, you can wear it, and you can eat it. You can make sails or fishing nets from it. You can treat burns and boils, wrap mummies, and prevent cancer with it. What is this wonder plant? Flax. For more than 10,000 years, man has been using flax to improve his health and his way of life.

Besides adding a great nutty flavor to your menu, you'll want to start eating flax for other reasons, too. It's a rich source of protein; essential fatty acids; vitamins; minerals, especially potassium; fiber; and phytoestrogens. It works equally well whether you take it as a supplement or get it in food. And the best news is, it can help protect your heart in several ways.

Puts the brakes on atherosclerosis. Compare your body to a car. Smoothly flowing oil keeps your car running better and longer. Smoothly flowing blood keeps your body running by reducing the likelihood of blood clots and keeping your heart from working so hard.

Just like the oil in your car, your blood tends to get thicker and stickier with age. While you can't run to the nearest quick-change shop and get a fresh supply of blood, adding a little flaxseed to your diet may be the next best thing. That's because flaxseed is the best vegetable source of omega-3 fatty acids. Omega-3 helps keep your blood from becoming sticky, which lowers your risk of heart attack and stroke.

When you think of omega-3 fatty acids, you may think of fish, since many varieties are high in this important nutrient. But sometimes getting enough fish or fish oil in your diet is hard. If that's the case, flaxseed is an easy, smart way to supplement. For more information on omega-3 fatty acids, see the *Fish and fish oil* chapter.

In addition to omega-3, flax is important because it contains lignan, an antioxidant. This means it works hard to destroy free radicals that can lead to atherosclerosis.

Helps control cholesterol. Give thanks for your daily bread — it may be getting rid of all that bad, artery-clogging cholesterol, especially if it's flaxseed bread. It's a proven fact that fiber in grains, like flax, helps lower your bad LDL cholesterol, and it may even raise your good HDL cholesterol. In addition, fiber really fills you up, leaving less room for meats, eggs, and dairy products that are high in cholesterol and fats.

One study found that when people with high cholesterol ate six slices of flaxseed bread a day, their cholesterol levels dropped significantly, even compared with those who ate six slices of wheat bread. If that sounds like too much bread for you, consider this.

After testing different amounts and types of flaxseed products, researchers at the University of Toronto came to the conclusion that up to 50 grams of flaxseed a day is safe and beneficial. They discovered this amount of raw flaxseed, flaxseed flour, or even flaxseed oil lowered LDL cholesterol by as much as 18 percent.

To profit from flax's heart-saving benefits, try to get 50 grams or about 1.5 ounces in your diet every day. Remember, it doesn't all have to come in one sitting, or from one type of product.

Adding flax to your diet is easy

Flaxseed may seem like a strange food to you, but there are many different and delicious ways to include it in your diet.

Add a few tablespoons of flaxseed for crunch and a nutty flavor in cookies, breads, and muffins. Sprinkle some in your salads and soups. Stir a spoonful into your orange juice or use it to top off your hot or cold cereal.

You can buy flaxseed flour or make your own by grinding the seeds in a blender or coffee grinder. Substitute it for regular flour when you're baking almost anything, like muffins, breads, cakes, or pancakes. Try using it as a thickener when making sauces. Add a bit to some water and you have a fat-free egg substitute for baked goods.

Try using flaxseed oil the next time you stir-fry. It will add a unique taste. But be aware that the oil becomes rancid quickly, so it's probably a good idea to buy small amounts at a time and make sure you store it properly. Read the labels since many flaxseed products should be refrigerated, or at least stored in a cool, dry place.

Although the fiber in flax is a big plus for your heart, it can cause gas if your body is not used to it. Start by adding flax to your diet gradually. A mere 3 ounces of flaxseed contains about 28 grams of fiber.

If you have any health problems, talk with your doctor before adding flaxseed to your diet.

🐾 🐾 🐾

The makings of a better chicken

Chickens fed a diet high in flax not only lay eggs with a higher content of alpha-linolenic acid, an omega-3 fatty acid your body needs for even the most basic functions, but the chicks born to them have less cholesterol in their own liver tissues.

🐾 🐾

Fruitful Flaxseed Bread

1 cup ground flaxseed
2 cups all-purpose flour
1 cup whole wheat flour
1/2 teaspoon vanilla extract
1 teaspoon salt
1 teaspoon baking soda
1 teaspoon baking powder
1 teaspoon cinnamon
egg substitute (equivalent to 2 eggs)
1 cup whole milk with 1 tablespoon of vinegar added (let it sit for 5 minutes)
juice and grated peel from two lemons
1/2 cup sugar
2 cups raisins, soaked in water

Preheat oven to 375 degrees F. Grease muffin cups or small (3x7-inch) loaf pans. Mix flour and ground flaxseed in a large bowl. Add raisins to dry mixture. Add vanilla, egg substitute, milk and vinegar, and lemon juice together to equal 1 1/2 cups. Combine liquid and dry mixtures. Stir just until blended. Pour batter into greased baking pans (approximately 2/3 full).

Bake for 15 to 20 minutes for muffins and 35 to 40 minutes for loaves.

Makes 20 to 24 servings

Per serving: 165 Calories; 5g Fat (0g from saturated fat) (26% calories from fat); 5g Protein; 27g Carbohydrate; 1mg Cholesterol; 172mg Sodium

Garlic

4 reasons to eat more garlic

Picture a rubber band that's been sitting in a drawer for a few years. It's no longer soft and stretchy but has turned hard and cracks easily. Now picture your arteries. They begin life just like that rubber band, soft and stretchy. But as you get older, they become stiff and inflexible — simply a natural part of aging. Only now this stiffness means every time your heart beats, your arteries don't spring back as easily as they used to, and you can end up with high blood pressure. Blood doesn't flow as smoothly through these stiffened arteries either, which causes a buildup of fats, leading to atherosclerosis. That means a greater chance of a heart attack or stroke.

Here's where garlic comes in. This small, unassuming herb, which has been used in cooking and healing for thousands of years, can put that spring back into your arteries — and your life. Researchers in Germany found that garlic pills kept the main artery to the heart soft and flexible. In fact, the older the test volunteers were, the greater the benefit.

Although researchers are still studying exactly how garlic works this minor miracle, they do know it improves blood flow in your arteries, keeping them, and your heart, strong and healthy. But garlic doesn't stop there. It contributes to your health in several other ways.

Blasts away blood clots. Research has proven that garlic makes your blood less sticky, less likely to clot. Fewer clots mean a lower chance of heart attack and stroke. But to get this heart-saving advantage, you need to take low doses over a long period of time. An occasional high dose just doesn't do the trick. Make garlic an everyday part of your cooking style and stop blood clots before they start.

Shields your arteries. If you've read anything at all about antioxidants, you know flavonoids provide powerful protection against artery damage. Nutritionists were thrilled to discover these natural disease-fighting compounds in many fruits and vegetables, as well as garlic.

Conquers cholesterol. Several recent studies claim there is no hard evidence that garlic lowers cholesterol. There are, however, dozens of past studies declaring just the opposite — that garlic prevents the build up of fat and cholesterol in your arteries, reduces triglycerides, and increases HDL cholesterol. In one of those studies, eating a fresh clove of garlic every day for 16 weeks reduced cholesterol by an amazing 20 percent.

Since garlic has been proven healthy in so many other ways, you can't go wrong adding it to your menu. In fact, if cholesterol is a concern for you, plan a few meals around garlic and fatty fish, like salmon. This combination seems to lower cholesterol better than either one alone. See the *Fish and fish oil* chapter for more information on fish high in omega-3 fatty acids.

Boycotts high blood pressure. If you need to get those blood pressure numbers down, don't despair. Garlic is best known for loosening up those arteries and allowing the blood to flow more easily. This means less stress on your heart and better circulation. Some studies suggest garlic can lower blood pressure by several points.

All these studies tested various forms of garlic — garlic powder, garlic extract, and garlic oil, as well as garlic cloves. Although experts aren't saying if you get more benefit from fresh garlic over garlic supplements, most nutritionists agree it's a good idea to use whole foods whenever possible. Supplements can be missing vital, health-saving benefits found only in a whole food.

If you are trying to figure out equal amounts, one clove of garlic is about the same as 1,000 milligrams (mg) of a garlic supplement.

Onions — another weapon against heart disease

The ancient Egyptians considered the onion a symbol of eternity. This nutritious bulb promises good health because of its vitamin C, fiber, and mineral content. In addition, onions add flavor to almost any dish without adding calories, fat, or salt. And as if that wasn't enough, they are a delicious weapon in the war on heart disease.

A mere half a cup of raw onion contains over 125 milligrams (mg) of potassium, a mineral proven to treat and prevent high blood pressure. In one study, a potassium-rich diet led to a 36 percent reduction in the use of high blood pressure medication. Apparently, it works by stimulating the body to get rid of excess salt and to release helpful hormones and chemicals into the bloodstream.

Onions also contain flavonoids, naturally occurring antioxidants. Flavonoids help keep your LDL cholesterol from joining with oxygen and damaging your artery walls. They also reduce the tendency of your blood to clot. Studies have shown that people with very low intakes of flavonoids have a higher risk of developing heart disease.

The particular flavonoid in onions, called quercetin, seems to be absorbed especially well by the digestive system. In tests, quercetin took about three hours to reach peak amounts in the bloodstream, and then levels dropped off again after the second day.

To get the greatest amount of quercetin, choose darker colored onions. Red contain the most, while white onions contain little, if any, of this heart-saving element.

Pasta Blasta

8 ounces bow-tie pasta
2 teaspoons margarine or olive oil
2 teaspoons minced garlic from a jar*
1 medium onion, sliced
1 pound boneless, skinless chicken breasts, cut into bite-sized pieces
3 tablespoons Dijon mustard
2 tablespoons honey
1/2 cup low-sodium chicken or vegetable broth
2 cups frozen vegetable medley (stir-fry blend, for example)
salt and pepper
grated Parmesan cheese to garnish

Cook pasta according to package directions, drain, and set aside.

Meanwhile, heat margarine or olive oil in a non-stick pan on medium-high heat and add garlic, onion, and chicken. Cook until chicken browns and is cooked through, about 10 to 12 minutes. Remove chicken from pan and set aside.

Add mustard and honey to pan; gradually stir in broth and bring mixture to a simmer.

Add frozen vegetables to pan, cover, and cook about 6 minutes, until vegetables are warmed.

Add cooked chicken, and salt and pepper to taste.

Serve chicken and vegetables over pasta and garnish with cheese if desired.

Available at grocery stores, usually in the produce section. You can use 2 crushed cloves of garlic if you prefer.

Makes 4 servings

Per serving: 487 Calories; 6g Fat (1g from saturated fat) (11% calories from fat); 40g Protein; 70g Carbohydrate; 66mg Cholesterol; 480mg Sodium

This is an official 5 A Day Recipe. This recipe is provided by the National Institutes of Health.

White Bean Pâté

This spread resembles the wonderfully aromatic French boursin cheese, but contains much less fat.

1/2 cup minced scallions
3 cloves garlic, minced
15 ounces canned white beans (navy or cannelini)
2 teaspoons Dijon mustard
1 tablespoon fresh lemon juice
1 teaspoon olive oil
2 tablespoons minced parsley
1 tablespoon minced basil
1 teaspoon minced thyme leaves

1 teaspoon minced dill
1 teaspoon minced tarragon
1/4 teaspoon nutmeg
salt and freshly ground pepper to taste

Combine all ingredients in a blender or food processor. Process until smooth.

Serve with crackers or pita bread.

Makes 12 servings

Per serving: 50 Calories; 1g Fat (less than 1g from saturated fat) (10% calories from fat); 3g Protein; 9g Carbohydrate; 0mg Cholesterol; 14mg Sodium

American Diabetes website: www.diabetes.org
Book ordering number 1-800-232-6733

Reprinted with permission of the American Diabetes Association, from Flavorful Seasons Cookbook, by K. Spicer. ©1996.

Roasted Onion Confiture

As an appetizer, this recipe is delicious served on top of garlic toast. You can also serve it with fish, beef, or chicken breasts.

2 (about 1 pound total) sweet onions (such as Vidalia), chopped
2 teaspoons olive oil
1/4 teaspoon salt
1/4 teaspoon freshly ground pepper
3 tablespoons raisins
1 tablespoon + 1 teaspoon balsamic vinegar
2 teaspoons drained capers

Preheat oven to 350 degrees F.

In a mixing bowl, toss onions with oil, salt, and pepper. Prepare flat baking pan with cooking spray. Spread onions on the pan.

Cover with foil and bake 30 minutes. Turn onions; bake uncovered another 15 minutes until onions are tender and begin to brown.

Stir in raisins, vinegar, and capers. Put into small container and refrigerate several hours before using, to allow flavors to blend.

Makes 8 servings, about 2 cups

Per serving: 32 Calories; 1g Fat (0g from saturated fat) (32% calories from fat); 1g Protein; 5g Carbohydrate; 0mg Cholesterol; 284mg Sodium

Reprinted with permission from The Art of Cooking for the Diabetic by Mary Abbott Hess, 1996

Germ Warfare

Antibiotics for heart disease — miracle cure or false hope?

Could a microscopic organism attack your arteries, much like a cold germ invades your sinuses, and cause heart disease? And, more importantly, could the cure for heart disease be as simple as an antibiotic? Ever since the bacteria *Helicobacter pylori* was discovered to cause ulcers, the possibility of linking bacteria to other conditions, such as heart disease, has intrigued scientists.

A bacterial cause would certainly explain the cycle of heart disease occurrences from 1940 to 1970. Scientists say the rise and fall in numbers is strangely similar to that of an infectious epidemic.

Researchers are investigating the theory that *Chlamydia pneumoniae*, bacteria that cause sinusitis, bronchitis, and pneumonia, may also damage arterial walls. This damage eventually leads to a buildup of cholesterol or an increase in blood clots, both risk factors for heart disease.

Scientists took notice of this theory when they were studying a group of people suffering from atherosclerosis.

They found that more than 73 percent had *C. pneumoniae* bacteria in the arteries of their heart. Only 4 percent of the group without atherosclerosis had evidence of the bacteria. In another study, total cholesterol was higher and good HDL cholesterol was lower in those suffering from this type of infection.

In an effort to test this theory, researchers in Utah infected rabbits with *C. pneumoniae*. The animals' major blood vessels thickened considerably. Those treated with an antibiotic had no thickening.

The research results are fascinating, but not entirely convincing. There is still no direct evidence that a bacterial infection actually causes specific types of heart disease, like atherosclerosis, although scientists have found certain bacteria at the site of artery damage.

Coincidence or cause? Whatever the explanation, many researchers believe a recent bacterial infection may be a risk factor for heart attack, especially in people over the age of 50.

Brush and floss to prevent a heart attack

Would you like to cut your risk of heart disease? Then brush your teeth.

Bacteria thrive in your mouth, and they like living in your gums. If you have sores from gum disease, it's an open invitation for bacteria to enter your bloodstream. Once there, the bacteria cause more inflammation, which can trigger your blood to clot and cause a heart attack.

When a prestigious medical journal reported on a study where dental health was significantly worse in people suffering heart attacks, scientists began to look for hard evidence of a link between gum disease and heart disease. What they found could be the answer to this relationship.

Researchers took bacteria from the mouths of people with gum disease. They were particularly interested in a common bacteria, *Porphyromanas gingivalis*. When they put the bacteria in a blood sample, the blood began to clump together. Because millions of people suffer from gum disease caused by this bacteria, they may be at risk of developing heart disease if it travels from their mouths into their bloodstreams. The type of clumping they observed in the laboratory could mean blocked arteries and strokes in humans.

Some experts are still not convinced that one condition causes the other. They say gum disease and heart disease may just be associated — people who don't take care of their teeth may not care about other aspects of their health. Still, a study of almost 10,000 people showed a 25 percent increased risk of heart disease in those with gum disease.

What you need to do is play it safe and take extra care of your teeth and gums. Brush twice a day, floss daily, and get regular dental checkups. If you develop any of these problems — tooth decay, root abscesses, tooth infection, tooth loss, and loss of supporting bone — you may have gum disease. For your heart's sake, see your dentist.

And one final point, smokers are five times more likely to suffer from gum disease. One more reason to kick the habit.

🐛 🐛 🐛

The germ that's not just for ulcers anymore

There may be more bacteria at work behind heart disease than first thought. A recent British study questioned if *Helicobacter pylori*, the same bacteria that causes ulcers, is also a risk factor for stroke. What researchers found is that people who had *H. pylori* antibodies in their blood also had greater narrowing of their carotid arteries than those who didn't. This is a major indicator of stroke.

The good news — an antibiotic that rids your stomach of *H. pylori* and ulcers could do the same for your heart.

🐛 🐛

Ginkgo

Ancient Chinese remedy enhances heart health

The maidenhair tree sounds like it should appear in a fairy tale, but you probably know it as ginkgo or even ginkgo biloba. It's the world's oldest living type of tree. A single ginkgo can live an astonishing 1,000 years, immune to the effects of pollution, pests, and disease. Add to that the healing properties of the ginkgo's leaf extract, and you truly have the stuff of fairy tales.

Chinese herbalists have been using ginkgo for various ailments since 2800 B.C. However, it wasn't until the 20th century that modern scientists accepted ginkgo into the approved stock of herbal medicine.

Today, a standard concentrated form, called ginkgo biloba extract (GBE), is used to treat Raynaud's disease, which causes poor circulation in the hands and feet; destroy free-radicals; improve memory; and relieve dizziness, asthma, and heart problems, among other things. Most studies use this extract and not the ground up leaf. Be aware that the two products may give you completely different results. In health studies on ginkgo, researchers most often used 40 milligrams (mg) three times a day. Experts say you will probably have to take the supplements for four to six weeks before you notice any difference in your health.

There are generally no side effects from ginkgo, but if you experience diarrhea, nausea, vomiting, or restlessness, either reduce the amount of GBE you are taking, stop altogether, or see a doctor.

5 ways ginkgo can increase longevity

Guards against blood clots. Ginkgo helps keep your blood from clumping together. A lower risk of blood clots means a lower risk of heart attack and stroke. If you are already taking a blood thinner or anticoagulant, talk to your doctor before you supplement with ginkgo.

Boosts circulation. If you've got a blood flow problem, ginkgo may be just the herb for you. Sluggish blood can cause plaque buildup, the first step in developing atherosclerosis. Numerous studies have proven that ginkgo can relax and widen your arteries, allowing better circulation throughout your body. Wider blood vessels could also mean lower blood pressure.

Acts as an antioxidant. Ginkgo helps keep LDL cholesterol from joining with oxygen and causing damage to the walls of your arteries.

Strikes at strokes. Ginkgo is especially helpful in getting more blood and oxygen flowing to your brain. This could help prevent strokes and their damage.

Cuts your cholesterol. In one study, a combination of garlic and ginkgo reduced total cholesterol levels by as much as 10 percent.

Grapes and Red Wine

A grape way to prevent heart attacks

You may have heard that drinking alcohol can help prevent heart attacks. But if alcoholic beverages aren't usually in your cupboard, don't rush out to the package store.

Wine or grape juice may help your heart independently of alcohol. The reason for this is in the processing of the grapes. To make white wine, the skins are removed from the grapes. But the skins are left on when making red wine. Could grape skins have something special that helps fight heart disease? Research confirms that grape skins contain two very important elements: flavonoids and resveratrol.

Flavonoids provide your body with powerful antioxidant protection. This means they control the amount of bad LDL cholesterol that combines with oxygen, which can damage your artery walls. Flavonoids can also increase the amount of good cholesterol in your body and help prevent blood clots. In addition to grape skins, nutritionists were thrilled to discover these natural disease-fighting compounds in many other fruits, vegetables, and herbs, such as strawberries, apples, grapefruit, onions, garlic, and ginger.

Resveratrol is a type of plant estrogen, or phytoestrogen. It works in your body by fighting inflammation, preventing blood clots, and reducing your risk of cancer.

Drinking moderate amounts of red wine — two to three glasses a day for healthy men and one to two glasses a day for healthy women — can indeed decrease your risk of heart disease. However, you don't have to drink alcohol to enjoy this healthy effect.

Although red grape juice contains only about half as many flavonoids as red wine, and they aren't as easily absorbed, it can give you similar antioxidant and phytoestrogen protection. In addition, about 12 ounces a day will not only help keep your blood from clumping together, it will give you a healthy dose of vitamins and minerals.

See the *Alcohol* chapter for more information about heart health and wine, beer, and liquor.

Grapes with Orange Zest

This recipe makes a pretty and simple dessert when served in a small glass dish and is equally nice as a fruit with breakfast or on a buffet.

1 navel orange
1/2 pound seedless red grapes
1/2 pound seedless green grapes
1 tablespoon chopped fresh mint leaves, (optional)

Remove 2 teaspoons zest from orange, using a zester or fine grater. Squeeze juice from orange into a 1-quart refrigerator container. Stir in zest.

Wash grapes and remove stems. If grapes are large, cut them in half. Put grapes into container with orange juice. Cover and shake to marinate grapes. Add mint if desired.

If time permits, refrigerate at least 1 hour for flavors to blend.

Makes 4 servings

Per serving: 58 Calories; less than 1g Fat (0g from saturated fat) (3% calories from fat); 1g Protein; 15g Carbohydrate; 0mg Cholesterol; 7mg Sodium

Reprinted with permission from The Art of Cooking for the Diabetic by Mary Abbott Hess, 1996

Guar Gum

High-fiber additive blasts cholesterol

Gums are a form of soluble fiber that pass through your system without being digested. They are called gums because when mixed with liquid they become thick and gel-like. A common example is guar gum.

The guar plant, grown in East India and Pakistan, produces a cluster bean called the guar seed. When the inner seed is dried and ground into a powder, the resulting guar gum is used as a thickening agent, like cornstarch. Guar gum is also added to foods and drugs to improve texture, bind various ingredients together, and improve the stability of many products. You can find it in everything from soft drinks to baked goods to salad dressings.

Recent research indicates that guar gum also can help reduce cholesterol levels by moving food rapidly through your digestive system. It's possible it could also affect the cholesterol-binding action of bile. In fact, guar gum is one of only a few sources of fiber that has repeatedly been shown to reduce cholesterol. Others are pectin, psyllium, and oat bran.

A scientific study showed a 16 percent reduction in cholesterol in seven healthy volunteers who were fed 36 grams of guar seed for two weeks, in addition to their normal diet. Another group of volunteers enjoyed an 11 percent drop in cholesterol after two weeks of eating 15 grams of guar per day.

Further studies also show that adding gums to the diet can reduce LDL cholesterol by as much as 26 percent.

Don't be misled by its strange sounding name. Guar gum is a completely natural product, similar to wheat flour, arrowroot, and cornstarch. Adding gum to processed food, such as ice cream, is just like adding cornstarch to pudding. You can find guar gum in most health food stores.

Beware the guar gum diet pill

Some over-the-counter diet pills containing mostly guar gum make outrageous claims of fast and easy weight loss. The theory is that when taken with water, the pills swell to many times their original size, causing your stomach to feel full. The problem is these pills can also swell up in your intestines, esophagus, and throat. Several people have been hospitalized with throat blockages. One died.

Guar gum is present in foods in small, safe amounts. Concentrated pills are not the same. There are better ways to lose weight.

Herbs

5 herbs that improve heart health

Using plants for medicine is nothing new. In fact, many modern medicines were originally created from plants. Digitalis, long used in the treatment of heart failure, first came from the dried leaf of the foxglove plant.

Even though herbs can provide natural and inexpensive health protection, talk with your doctor before taking any herbs. Some herbs can interact with medication.

Hawthorn. This tree with its bright-red fruit is the heavy hitter of herbal heart therapy. Commonly called Mayblossom, its scientific name is *Crataegus oxyacantha*, which comes from the Greek words for "hardness," "sharp," and "thorn." It is related to the rose family, and its white flowers and scarlet fruit make it a popular ornamental tree.

Hawthorn contains flavonoids, which may be responsible for its heart-protecting effect. Flavonoids are known for their antioxidant activity. Extracts of hawthorn dilate blood vessels around your heart, resulting in a better supply of blood, oxygen, and nutrients. Hawthorn also reduces cholesterol levels and helps prevent cholesterol from sticking to your artery walls.

In Europe, hawthorn is used as a treatment for congestive heart failure. A recent study in Germany found that people with heart failure who took hawthorn extract improved their stamina and endurance and had lower blood pressure during exercise. Their hearts also pumped more blood at a lower pressure.

The German Commission E, which governs the use and sale of herbs in Germany, approves hawthorn for treatment of mild heart failure and a slow and irregular heartbeat.

In Europe and Asia, hawthorn is available by prescription, but you can buy hawthorn in the United States in health food and herb stores. It comes as a tincture or extract, or you can buy the dried berries and leaves to make teas.

Hawthorn takes a while to begin working. Experts say it takes at least two weeks before it has an effect. Taking large doses of hawthorn can be toxic. Check with your doctor before using.

Fenugreek. The name of this aromatic plant means "Greek hay." The seeds have a slightly sweet flavor, similar to maple sugar, and are used to flavor many foods, including imitation maple syrup. The seeds may also help lower your cholesterol and control your blood sugar.

A recent study of diabetics, who are more than twice as likely to die of heart disease than people who don't have diabetes, confirmed that fenugreek lowers cholesterol and blood sugar levels. Another study found that LDL (bad) cholesterol, VLDL (very bad) cholesterol, and triglycerides decreased steadily over a 24-week period. HDL (good) cholesterol increased by 10 percent over the same time period.

Fenugreek is high in fiber, which may account in part for its cholesterol-lowering effect. The seeds are available either whole or ground for use in cooking, or you can buy capsules at a health food store.

Ginseng. When you think of ginseng, you may think "aphrodisiac." Although ginseng's reputation for increasing sexual desire may be deserved, it has many other claims to improving health. In addition to increasing energy, improving blood sugar levels, and helping prevent certain types of cancer, ginseng may also be good for your heart.

Ginseng contains antioxidants, which can fight the effects of free radicals that damage your cells and arteries. Ginseng also contains a substance called sitosterol, which is absorbed by your intestines and lowers cholesterol. Several studies have found that ginseng lowers cholesterol in animals and may protect against brain damage from stroke.

If you decide to take ginseng supplements, read the label carefully to make sure you're getting the real thing. Some supplements contain very little ginseng. A quality ginseng product will contain ginsenosides. The more ginsenosides a product has, the more likely you'll benefit from it. Look for a product labeled "standardized" and one that contains 4 to 7 percent ginsenosides.

If you have high blood pressure, check with your doctor before taking it. Ginseng may raise blood pressure levels. Diabetics should also consult their doctors before taking ginseng because it lowers blood sugar levels.

Ginger. The gingerbread man from the famous children's story may have been able to run away from all those people because ginger kept his heart going strong. As an addition to tasty breads and cookies, ginger has been around a long time, but its use as a medicine goes back even farther. Ancient Chinese sailors used it as a remedy for motion sickness, and the ancient Greeks used it as a digestive aid.

Ginger is still going strong today, both as a spice and a health aid. Ginger is a powerful antioxidant, and it also helps keep your platelets from sticking together and forming clots. Numerous studies have confirmed this effect. One study found that 5 grams of ginger daily significantly inhibits platelets' ability to clump, which reduces the risk of clogged arteries in people with heart disease. Less blood clotting means less risk of a heart attack.

Ginger also may help lower cholesterol levels by improving your digestion of fats. Ginger does this by aiding the liver and gallbladder in their production and transportation of bile to the intestines where it helps your body digest fat.

The German Commission E recommends 2 to 4 grams daily to aid digestion and ease nausea. A similar dose might be helpful for your heart. Just adding some to your recipes now and then might spice them up, but it won't be enough for any substantial health benefits. You probably don't want to swallow a spoonful of the dry spice, either. That can cause an unpleasant burning in your mouth and throat. However, you can buy powdered ginger in gelatin capsules. Normally, you get 500 milligrams (mg) of powdered ginger per capsule. In order to get 2 to 4 grams of ginger, you'll need to take four to eight capsules.

Although ginger is safe for most people, ask your doctor before taking it if you:
- have gallstones.
- are pregnant.
- take heart medicine. Ginger may intensify the effects of heart drugs, which can be dangerous.
- are scheduled for surgery. Ginger's anti-clotting properties may cause you to bleed excessively.

Valerian. Are you wearing your heart out because you never relax? If you're nervous, tense, and can't seem to get a good night's sleep, this herb may be the key to calming you down and helping you slumber soundly.

Valerian has been used as a tranquilizer and relaxant for over 1,000 years. Modern studies have found it can significantly improve the quality of sleep. Although its name is similar to Valium, the brand name of a potent synthetic tranquilizer, valerian works much more gently. And, it doesn't carry the risk of addiction like many prescription sedatives. There is also little danger of overdosing on valerian.

Valerian may also help lower blood pressure, at least according to animal studies. If it doesn't lower it directly, it may help lower it indirectly by helping reduce your stress level.

The most commonly used form of valerian is a tincture. Herbal experts recommend dropping at least one teaspoonful into a glass of water or dissolving it on a sugar cube. They say you can take this dose every 15 to 30 minutes, up to three times a day. You can also make a soothing cup of valerian tea by adding two teaspoonfuls of the dried root to a cup of hot water.

More herbs for good health

Herb	Scientific name	Use
Bran	*Triticum aestivum*	Increases dietary fiber
Chamomiles and yarrow	*Matricaria recutita* *Chamaemelum nobile* *Achillea millefolium*	Aids digestion, inflammation, infections, minor illnesses
Chicory	*Cichorium intybus*	Calming, caffeine-free beverage
Evening primrose	*Oenothera biennis*	Lowers blood pressure
Fenugreek	*Trigonella foenum-graecum*	Lowers cholesterol and blood sugar
Garlic and other alliums	*Allium sativum* (garlic) *Allium cepa* (onion) *Allium ascalonicum* (scallion)	Improves atherosclerosis, lowers high blood pressure, lowers cholesterol
Ginger	*Zingiber officinale Roscoe*	Digestive aid, antiplatelet, lowers cholesterol
Gingko	*Gingko biloba*	Dilates blood vessels, improves blood flow

Herb	Scientific name	Use
Gingseng and related herbs	*Panax ginseng* (Oriental ginseng) *Panax quinquefolius* (American ginseng)	Relieves stress, improves memory, increases energy, lowers cholesterol
Hawthorn	*Crateagus laevigata*	Dilates blood vessels, strengthens heart, improves high blood pressure
Valerian	*Valeriana officinalis*	Calms nerves, aids sleep, relieves stress

Beware: These herbs may raise blood pressure

Herb	Scientific name	Use
Caffeine-containing plants: Coffee Tea Kola Cacao	*Coffea arabica* *Camellia sinensis* *Cola nitida* *Theobroma cacao*	Stimulant
Ephedra (Ma huang)	*Ephedra*	Anti-asthmatic, nasal decongestant
Licorice	*Glycyrrhiza glabra*	Treats coughs and colds
Mistletoe, American	*Phoradendron leucarpum*	Increases blood pressure
Rosemary	*Rosmarinus officinalis*	Stimulant

Curry Powder

The Chinese mustard and cayenne pepper are hot. You may want to decrease these ingredients or eliminate them altogether if you prefer less spiciness.

2 tablespoons ground coriander
2 tablespoons ground cumin
2 tablespoons ground ginger
2 tablespoons ground fenugreek
1 tablespoon dry Chinese hot mustard (optional)
2 teaspoons ground cayenne pepper (optional)
1/4 teaspoon crushed saffron
1 tablespoon horseradish powder

Sift all ingredients except saffron together. Sifting eliminates little clumps and evenly distributes all the powders. Add crushed saffron, mix thoroughly, and store in a tightly sealed glass jar.

Makes about 10 tablespoons

Per tablespoon: 19 Calories; 1g Fat (27% calories from fat); 1g Protein; 3g Carbohydrate; 0mg Cholesterol; 6mg Sodium

Three-Pepper Hazelnut Soup

1 quart chicken stock
1 cup lentils
1/2 cup chopped onions
1/2 cup chopped carrots

1/4 cup chopped celery
2 garlic cloves
1/2 teaspoon coriander
1/2 teaspoon fenugreek
1/4 teaspoon cumin
2 cups water
1 1/2 cups Hazelnuts, toasted and chopped
1 teaspoon mixed peppercorns (pink, green and black, cracked)
2 tablespoons roux: (equal parts soft butter and all-purpose flour worked into smooth paste)
sour cream, chopped onions, chives, shredded carrots, or Hazelnuts for garnish

Combine stock, lentils, onions, carrots, celery, garlic, coriander, fenugreek, and cumin in a heavy 3-quart soup pot.

Bring to boil, reduce heat and simmer 1 hour.

Remove from heat and put through a sieve, or puree and return to pot.

Add water, Hazelnuts, and 3 peppers and simmer 15 minutes.

Beat in roux to thicken and cook an additional 15 minutes. Salt to taste, then garnish.

Makes 6 main dish servings, 12 first course servings

Per serving: 136 Calories; 7g Fat (2g from saturated fat) (43% calories from fat); 7g Protein; 13g Carbohydrate; 5mg Cholesterol; 285mg Sodium

Reprinted with permission from the Hazelnut Growers of Oregon
www.hazelnut.com/recipes/soup1.html

Rice and Peas Curry

3 cups cooked brown rice
1 cup cooked green peas
1/4 cup diced onion
1/4 teaspoon salt
1 tablespoon curry powder (or to taste)
1/2 cup chicken broth

Combine all ingredients and microwave in a covered container on medium 3 to 4 minutes or until heated through and onions are translucent. Serve with a fresh green salad.

Makes 2 main dish servings, 4 to 6 side dish servings

Per serving: 376 Calories; 3g Fat (less than 1g from saturated fat) (7% calories from fat); 10g Protein; 77g Carbohydrate; 0mg Cholesterol; 225mg Sodium

Kiwifruit Shrimp Salad

1/2 pound California kiwifruit, pared and sliced
1/2 pound (21-30 size) shrimp, shelled, deveined and cooked with tails intact
1/2 cup finely julienned radish
1/2 cup finely julienned pomegranate
1/2 head butter lettuce

Lemon Ginger Dressing:

2 tablespoons olive oil
2 tablespoons vinegar

2 tablespoons lemon juice
1 tablespoon honey
1 teaspoon grated ginger
1/2 teaspoon salt
1/8 teaspoon pepper

Combine dressing ingredients and mix well. Makes about 1/3 cup.

Arrange all other ingredients in shallow lettuce-lined salad bowl. Serve with Lemon Ginger Dressing.

Makes 3 to 4 servings

Per serving: 192 Calories; 8g Fat (1g from saturated fat) (37% calories from fat); 13g Protein; 18g Carbohydrate; 86mg Cholesterol; 361mg Sodium

Reprinted with permission from the California Kiwifruit Commission

Job Stress Solutions

Stress management lowers heart disease risk

Stress can make you sick. It can cause you to feel dizzy and have sweaty hands. It can give you a headache, a stomachache, or a backache. It can make your heart pound and your chest tighten.

Stress on the job is especially hazardous. It has been called a worldwide epidemic, causing workplace accidents, violence, absenteeism, employee turnover, and millions of dollars in disability. Not only can stress affect your ability to work, it can begin a vicious cycle of tension and negative thoughts that can land you in the hospital. And not just for an ulcer, either. The more stress you feel at your workplace, the higher your risk of developing heart disease and stroke.

In a study in Finland, men who reacted to job stress with a significant rise in blood pressure had the most plaque in their carotid arteries, the arteries in the neck that supply blood to the head. Another study showed that increasing workload also increased the levels of several blood-clotting factors.

If you work on a shift schedule, you might be doing a stress-filled number on your heart and never even know it. Compared to day workers, shift workers had higher levels of cholesterol and tended to carry more weight around their midsection, both heart disease risk factors. Stress can cause your arteries to narrow and rupture, if they are blocked; it can raise your blood pressure; and if you're a woman, it can lower your estrogen.

These are all serious ways stress can influence your health. But there is hope — in the form of stress management. If you suffer from heart disease, you might be able to reduce your risk of suffering a heart attack or having to undergo heart surgery by an amazing 74 percent simply by learning to handle your stress.

Learn how the experts win out over worry

Type	Description	Example	Benefits	Drawbacks
Emotion-focused coping style	Do things to make oneself feel better.	Tell yourself you can get through this.	You can always use it. It can make you feel better immediately.	It doesn't make problems go away.
Problem-focused coping style	Try to fix the problem.	Discuss a problem with a co-worker who you think is wrong.	Sometimes this method makes problems go away.	You can't make some problems go away no matter how hard you try.
Relation-ship-focused coping style	Handle other people's needs.	Discuss how you feel with someone you are angry with.	You may help yourself or someone else.	You can't change other people.

Used with permission from Clinical Tools, Inc., Internet address <http://206.31.218.3/stress/control.htm>

13 ways to control the bad effects of stress

◆ **Find out what's going on.** If you have information on what is happening around you, you will feel more in control.

◆ **Let your feelings out.** Whether it's a cut-back, a firing, or a promotion, you're going to feel stress. Holding emotions in will not allow you to move on to more positive feelings. Go ahead and express your sadness or anxiety.

◆ **Make time for play.** Don't sacrifice your leisure time. Don't work through lunch. Don't skip your family vacation. Don't give up your weekends. Don't come home later and later on workdays. If you take time to recharge your battery and get away from work-related responsibilities, you'll probably return to the job with more energy and enthusiasm than before.

◆ **Pay attention to your family.** Spend time with them and make sure they know how important they are. In turn, they'll give you the kind of emotional support you need to handle your stress.

◆ **Don't cling to the past.** Realize there will always be change and try not to let it make you uncomfortable.

◆ **Stay away from drugs and alcohol.** Relying on these for relief can ruin your health and your life. The headaches, nervousness, and irritability you may feel from a high-stress job are nothing compared to the horrors of an addiction.

◆ **Call on a friend.** Your co-workers and supervisors may be more supportive than you think. If not, look for emotional support outside your workplace.

◆ **Eat healthy.** Your body needs good, solid nourishment from healthy foods. Get plenty of fresh fruits and vegetables. Don't skip meals, overeat, or grab quick junk food.

- **Focus on the positive.** Search for the good in your life, your job, and your relationships.

- **Celebrate every success.** Instead of moaning and groaning about your failures, take the time to recognize when things are going right. Throw a party, go out to dinner, treat yourself to a shopping trip — do something special to celebrate your accomplishments.

- **Be realistic.** Setting unreasonable goals places unnecessary stress on yourself and increases your risk of failure.

- **Exercise regularly.** The best defense is a good offense. By building a strong body, you are giving yourself the best tools to fight the bad effects of stress.

- **Find a hobby.** Spending time doing something you enjoy will allow you to unwind and take your mind off anxieties. Having a hobby also gives you something to look forward to during your free time.

For more ways to help you fight stress, see the chapters on *Alexander technique, Anger arresters, Aromatherapy, Exercise, Movement therapy, and Relaxation.*

Stop the world — I want to get off

Some people hate roller coasters because the speed and direction are out of their control. Others love that free, flying feeling. If you are the kind that passes "The Speed Demon" by every time, could you change yourself enough to overcome your anxiety? Could you learn to ride it with your hands in the air and your eyes wide open? Or could you only enjoy it if you were driving?

How much control do you feel you have over your life? This could be a very important question if you want to avoid heart disease. Researchers in Britain found that workers in clerical and support positions, those with little or no control over their jobs, were much more likely to develop heart disease than executives, people who make many of their own work-related decisions.

If lack of control is stressing you out, you can either learn to view life as one big amusement park, sit back and enjoy the ride, or you can get yourself into a situation where you drive the roller coaster. Either way, think long and hard about the way you view your life and the amount of stress you feel because of it.

Here are some terms researchers use to describe different feelings of control:

If you view the world this way:	You think this way:
Internal	"I control what happens to me."
External	"The world controls what happens to me."
Global	"This event has huge effects."
Specific	"This event has limited effects."
Stable	"Things will always be like this."
Unstable	"Things can change."

Used with permission from Clinical Tools, Inc., Internet address <http://206.31.218.3/stress/control.htm>

Learn natural ways to cope to lower blood pressure

Not all people in high-stress jobs become sick from stress. This notion is so different from common belief that researchers studied air traffic controllers, a line of work well-known for its high stress, in an effort to find out how this happens. They discovered something interesting. The controllers didn't have higher than normal blood pressure.

One explanation is that people drawn to high-stress jobs or those that are successful in them have a special ability for handling stress. They may have the type of personality that allows tension to roll right off them, or they may have made certain coping techniques, like exercise or quality family time, a natural part of their lives. In any event, these people have instinctive ways to keep stress from affecting their bodies.

Another theory is that it's not necessarily the job stress that raises your blood pressure, it's the way you cope with that stress. If you feel frustrated all morning and indulge in a hamburger and fries for lunch, or come home from a hard day at the office and unwind with a few drinks, you're not doing your heart any good. The boss lays another deadline on you, so you sneak out for a cigarette break. Things like diet, drinking habits, smoking, and physical activity could be the real influences on your blood pressure.

The answer seems to lie within each person. It's just not possible to remove every bit of stress from your life, but if you learn healthy, natural ways to handle pressure, you might live a longer, happier life.

{🐌 🐌 🐌}

How your paycheck can turn the tables on tension

Do you feel you don't get the proper reward for all your hard work? Do you put in the effort and commitment but never see that pay raise or promotion? If so, you are twice as likely as others to develop heart disease.

One way scientists define job stress is a high amount of effort spent and a low amount of reward received. In the job place, most people define reward as income. And researchers have found that low income, even without the usual types of job stress, increases your risk of dying from heart disease.

One study took a cross-section of workers and measured the amount of plaque buildup in their arteries. Those under stress and receiving low pay had nearly twice the amount of buildup as those with low stress and higher pay. When stress levels were not taken into consideration, heart disease risk was still higher in those workers with lower income.

Since it seems the negative effects of your job seem to depend most on your income level, perhaps you need to go ahead and ask for that raise — for your heart's sake.

{🐌 🐌}

Legumes

Eat legumes and get a leg-up on cholesterol

Don't let the funny name scare you away. Legumes are not some strange vegetarian dish you'll never find in your grocery store. They are the inexpensive beans and peas you've been eating for years. You may call them beans, but technically they're legumes, a term that includes hundreds of seed-pod plants like split peas, black-eyed peas, lentils, peanuts, kidney beans, lima beans, and soybeans.

One of nature's very best inventions, legumes are full of complex carbohydrates, protein, iron, B vitamins, minerals, and fiber. They are low in fat and high in phytoestrogens, which are natural plant estrogens. But perhaps their greatest health gift to mankind is their ability to lower cholesterol.

Test after test has proven that adding legumes to a healthy diet can make your cholesterol really take a nose-dive. Researchers think legumes keep your bile acids from circulating through your intestines as freely as usual. Since cholesterol is the main ingredient in bile, if the cholesterol doesn't circulate, it can't be absorbed into your blood where it can cause artery damage.

It doesn't matter if you buy your legumes fresh or canned. You can get the same heart-saving benefit from either. Just realize that canned beans may contain more sodium. To cut back on the salt, rinse them before serving.

One legume you may have overlooked is the chickpea or garbanzo bean. Perhaps you've seen these round, somewhat crunchy beans on your favorite salad bar. They are also a major part of Mediterranean and Latin American diets. If you've enjoyed a garlicky dip called hummus at your favorite Lebanese restaurant, you've been eating pureed chickpeas with a little olive oil and flavoring added.

Try including legumes in several of your daily meals or snacks. By eating a few small servings throughout the day, you may lower your cholesterol more than with just one large serving. This will also get you in the habit of making legumes a natural part of your diet.

4 great reasons to eat more beans

Fiber. A high-fiber diet can help reduce your risk of atherosclerosis, a major cause of heart attacks and strokes. You can cut your risk of heart attack by 20 percent just by adding 10 grams of fiber a day to your diet.

Protein. You don't need a lot of protein. In fact, the recommended dietary allowance (RDA) for people over 50 years ranges from just 46 to 56 grams. Most people in North America get well over this amount. This is important because in the case of protein, more is not better. If you want to get the most benefit from the least amount of protein, think beans. Some studies have shown that if you switch just half your protein intake from meat sources to legume sources, you can lower your cholesterol by 10 percent or more.

Iron. This essential mineral keeps your blood cells running strong as they transport oxygen and other necessary materials throughout your body. Without enough iron, you have tired, sluggish blood cells and that means a tired, sluggish you — bad news for your heart.

Folic acid. Legumes are a great source of folic acid, which can lower your risk of heart attack and stroke. You can read more about this important member of the vitamin family in the *B vitamins* chapter.

The following table shows you just how much of these important nutrients you can find in several common types of legumes.

Type 1/2 cup, cooked	% of RDA for women over 50			
	Fiber	Protein	Folate	Iron
black beans	36	16	32	25
black-eyed peas	27	14	45	27
broadbeans	22	14	22	16
chickpeas	25	13	20	20
great northern beans	30	16	23	24
kidney beans	39	15	16	20
lentils	37	19	45	41
lima beans	31	16	20	28
mung beans	27	15	21	20
navy beans	28	17	32	28
pinto beans	33	17	37	22
soybeans	25	31	12	55
split peas	39	18	16	16
white beans	27	19	18	41

Easy ways to liven up your legumes

- Substitute beans for the ground beef in your favorite recipe.

- Toss some beans in your next green salad for added crunch and color.

- Make a sandwich or pita out of mashed, cooked beans, flavored with onions, celery, green peppers, garlic powder, or a ready-made salsa.

- Add them to any traditional soup recipe.

- Combine any type of legume with cold pasta and low-fat dressing for a light entree.

- Revive the old tradition of a baked bean supper.

- Make your own refried beans by mashing cooked beans with a little olive or canola oil and a bit of finely ground Canadian bacon.

- Don't make your baked beans or chili with the same old beans — experiment with different types and combinations.

- Buy ethnic cookbooks for terrific ways to use legumes in different ways.

Black Bean Soup

12 ounces black beans
1 lemon, peeled, sliced thick
1/2 medium onion, diced
1/4 teaspoon ground cumin
1 fresh jalapeno, seeded, minced
1 teaspoon dried marjoram leaves
2 teaspoons sherry wine vinegar
2 quarts chicken or vegetable broth, unsalted
1 slice bacon, diced
2 cloves garlic, minced
1 tablespoon chili powder

6 sun-dried tomatoes, chopped
1/2 tsp salt

Soak the beans overnight covered with water by 3 inches. Drain beans and simmer in stock with lemon slices until beans are tender.

In frying pan, cook bacon over medium heat until fat rendered; add onion and cumin; cook until onion is soft. Add onion mixture, garlic, chili powder, jalapeno, tomatoes, marjoram, and salt to the beans. Simmer 15 minutes.

Remove lemon. Remove 1/3 of the bean mixture; puree and return to soup. Add vinegar.

Makes 10 servings

Per serving: 226 Calories; 2g Fat (0g from saturated fat) (6% calories from fat); 21g Protein; 43g Carbohydrate; 1mg Cholesterol; 744mg Sodium

This is an official 5 A Day Recipe. This recipe provided by the National Institutes of Health.

Chickpea Dip with Vegetables

This healthier-than-hummus dip goes well with pita bread and is great for a party. It also provides one and a half servings of vegetables per serving.

1 can (12 1/2 ounces) chickpeas, drained and rinsed well
1 cup (8 ounce container) plain low-fat yogurt
2 tablespoons fresh lemon juice
1/2 tablespoon olive oil
3 drops hot pepper sauce
1 carrot, grated

2 cucumbers, peeled, seeded and diced
2 Roma tomatoes, finely chopped
1/4 red onion, diced

Blend chickpeas, yogurt, lemon juice, olive oil, and hot sauce in a blender until smooth.

Transfer dip to a shallow serving bowl and pile the colorful vegetables on top, leaving an outer rim of dip to be seen.

Serve with pita bread or toasted wheat bread triangles.

Makes 6 servings

Per serving: 278 Calories; 6g Fat (1g from saturated fat) (17% calories from fat); 15g Protein; 45g Carbohydrate; 2mg Cholesterol; 50mg Sodium

This is an official 5 A Day Recipe. This recipe is provided by the National Institutes of Health.

Low-fat Eating

Shake bad habits for lower blood pressure

High blood pressure increases your risk for many serious diseases, including heart disease, stroke, and kidney failure. Although most people rely on medication to control their blood pressure, many high blood pressure drugs may make you wonder if the cure is worse than the ailment. Among some of the reported side effects are headaches, poor appetite, upset stomach, dry mouth, diarrhea, stuffy nose, dizziness, and tingling or numbness in the hands or feet. It's comforting to know you have other choices.

One university study found that over 85 percent of the people with high blood pressure were able to stop taking their blood pressure medicine when they received dietary and lifestyle counseling, and took this counseling to heart. Not only that, after making the lifestyle changes, their blood pressure was actually lower than when they were on the drugs.

This important discovery was confirmed at the University of Minnesota. A study pitted three test groups against each other. One group stopped taking their blood pressure medicine and received nutritional counseling, a second group stopped taking it and received no counseling, and a third simply continued as normal. After four years, 40 percent of the first group were enjoying normal blood pressure without drugs, while 95 percent of those in groups two and three were on medicine.

The participants in these studies achieved and maintained their normal blood pressure by losing weight and eating foods low in fat.

The safest way to lower your blood pressure is to make lifestyle changes and work with your doctor. Don't stop taking any medication without checking with him first.

Learn the secrets to low-fat eating

A low-fat diet can reduce your total cholesterol level by as much as 12 percent. Of course, if you lose weight along with this change in your diet, you'll be doing your heart an even greater favor. The bad cholesterol will go down, and your good cholesterol won't be affected.

Fat has gotten a bad rap lately. In fact, many experts say all this fat panic is somewhat misguided. Your body cannot manage without fat. It is one of your best sources of energy, your cells need it to function properly, it is necessary for human growth, and it carries the fat-soluble vitamins, A, D, E, and K, throughout your body. And did you know that a little fat actually helps to curb your appetite? That's why a very low-fat diet may make you feel hungry all the time. Fat also makes food taste better. It allows you to experience all the flavors in food, and it adds a certain texture or "mouth feel" to them.

If you decide to cut back on fat, don't overdo it. Cutting your fat intake too much can actually do your heart more harm than good. One study showed that triglycerides went up and good HDL cholesterol levels went down on very low-fat diets — those containing only about 20 percent fat.

In addition, most people have what is called pattern A cholesterol. This means their LDL cholesterol is large and spread out. Others, though, have pattern B — small, dense, LDL cholesterol, which is the baddest of the bad. With pattern B, you are at an even higher risk of heart disease. Testing has shown that a very low-fat diet can shift those with pattern A to pattern B. That means they begin producing compact, dangerous LDL cholesterol. Although doctors are working on it, there is no easy test to find out which pattern you are.

The answer is to reduce the amount of fat in your diet by a reasonable amount. The U.S. Department of Agriculture and the U.S. Department of Health and Human Services recommend a total dietary fat intake of no more than 30 percent of your total calories. That means if you are on a 2,000 calorie-a-day diet, you should not eat more than 600 fat calories a day. And keep the saturated fat, found primarily in meat and dairy products, as low as possible. The American Heart Association says saturated fat should be no more than 7 percent of your total daily calories.

Don't get confused by all these numbers. Most food labels list the number of fat calories per serving. But if you want to figure out how much fat is in a certain food, you can simply do a little math. Here's how you can calculate the fat.

1. First, you need to know there are 9 calories in a gram of fat.

2. Check the food label to find out how many grams of fat are in a serving of the food item. Let's say 5, for example.

3. Multiply 9 x 5 to find out the number of calories from fat you will be eating. In this case, the number of calories is 45.

4. You can stop there or go on to figure out a percentage. Read the label for the number of calories per serving in your chosen food. Let's say it's 300.

5. Divide the fat calories (45) by the calories per serving (300) to get the percentage of calories from fat (15 percent) in that food.

If you're not the kind of person who likes to keep track of these things, simply cut out high-fat foods or substitute low-fat versions for them.

You'll find the less fat you eat, the less you'll crave it. In fact, one study found that people on a very low calorie diet showed the biggest drop in cravings. It should make you feel better to know that denying yourself certain foods doesn't make you want them more.

For more information on ways to replace fat in your diet, see the *Fat substitutes* chapter.

Think lean when choosing meat

If you've always been a meat and potatoes kind of person but decided to give meat the heave-ho for the sake of your low-fat diet, there's reason to rejoice. As long as you exercise a little control, it's OK to eat meat. In fact, some health experts think it's probably better than going totally meat-free.

If you give up on meat, you may be depriving yourself of more than just a favorite food. Lean meat is an important source of protein, vitamins, and minerals. Meat supplies lots of iron, which is particularly important to women and not very common in other foods. Elderly people sometimes need the extra zinc found in meat.

You may think meat is your main source of fat, but for most people, it only accounts for about one-fourth of their fat consumption. Did you know that one glazed doughnut contains more fat than 3 ounces of top sirloin? And although 70 percent of dietary cholesterol comes from the meat group, over half of that amount comes from eggs.

Instead of cutting meat out of your diet, select your cuts of meat carefully. Choose beef cuts with the words "loin" or "round" in the name. Pick "choice" instead of "prime" and choose cuts graded "USDA Select." When buying pork, pick cuts with the word "loin" or "leg" in the name.

Once you've chosen your meat carefully, trim away the excess fat, and use low-fat cooking methods, like broiling, steaming, baking, roasting, or grilling. If you're careful, you can maintain your low-fat diet and still enjoy a good steak now and then.

20 tasty ways to eat less fat

- Substitute small amounts of olive oil for butter and margarine.

- Use margarine made with liquid vegetable oil instead of butter.

- Buy turkey, a good low-fat choice, instead of other lunch meats.

- Use a nonstick skillet and a cooking spray instead of tablespoons of oil.

- Replace meat in your favorite recipes with beans or tofu.

- Use low-fat plain yogurt instead of sour cream.

- Chill soups and stews before eating and skim the solid fat off the top.

- Sprinkle herbs and spices on vegetables instead of drowning them in butter or cream sauces.

- Boost flavor without boosting fat by adding Dijon mustard, salsa, balsamic vinegar, or chili sauce to your dishes.

- Make your own salad dressing with more vinegar and less oil. Choose flavored vinegars or lemon juice for added zing.

- Replace butter or oil in baked goods with applesauce or prune puree. (See the *Fat substitutes* chapter for more information.)

- Microwave, steam, grill, broil, or sauté foods in stock.

- Remove skin and breaded coating from foods.

- Choose yeast breads, like English muffins and French bread, since they are more likely to be made without much fat.

- Don't add salt or oil to the water when cooking rice, pasta, or hot cereals — it's not necessary.

- Whip low-fat cottage cheese with a little lemon juice for a great baked potato topping.

- Baste your roasting meats with fruit juice or unsalted tomato juice rather than pan drippings.

- Cut back on the amount of cheese in your sauces and add a dash of dry mustard for flavor.

- Substitute undiluted evaporated milk for cream.

- Use part-skim mozzarella cheese instead of cheddar, Swiss, or processed American.

Tips for making a hero of a sandwich

There can be more fat grams lurking between two slices of bread than you might think. Here are some ways you can cut the fat and keep the flavor.

- **Consider going vegetarian.** If you avoid meat altogether, you can still have a hearty handful with practically no fat. Be creative. Shred some carrots, slice a cucumber, and pick some sprouts. Chop some celery and add peppers, beets, onions, or mushrooms. Practically anything you find in your produce aisle can go on a sandwich. Don't get in a lettuce rut, either. Spinach, chicory, and romaine are deliciously healthy alternatives.

- **Spread it thin.** Unless you choose a nonfat mayonnaise, you are heading into fat heaven with this popular dressing. Try a spread that's loaded with zip but not the fat, like mustard, ketchup, salsa, hummus, or even vinegar.

◆ **Say cheese, please.** Pick your cheese, carefully. A slice of Swiss can have up to 5 grams of saturated fat. Go for the nonfat or part-skim versions.

◆ **Give up high-fat meat.** You may have grown up on bologna, but now it's time to bid this fat-loaded lunch meat a fond farewell. Turkey is your best choice, even if you don't go for the fat-free variety. It's low in calories and naturally lean. Ham still remains the number one seller in most delis, but you really need to watch the sodium. Try one of the low-fat, low-sodium products at your grocer — you may never notice the taste difference. If you've got the time, the best solution is to cook your own white meat chicken or turkey, and keep it on hand for your next sandwich attack.

Eat the foods you love without betraying your heart

Do you adore cheesy lasagna, grilled cheese sandwiches, and macaroni and cheese? If so, you have lots of company. A recent study found that many women get most of their saturated fat from cheese. If you don't want to give up the foods you love, try some of the reduced-fat or fat-free varieties. While the reduced-fat versions can lower cholesterol, they contain about the same amount of calories as regular cheese. Fat-free cheese, on the other hand, is lower in both calories and fat.

And what about hamburgers. Do you crave the taste but hate the fat? If so, try this cooking method. Microwave your patties for one to three minutes; pour off the liquid; and then fry, broil, or grill them. This method cuts the fat content by almost one-third, and it has another benefit besides. Substances that may cause cancer are sometimes formed when cooking burgers at high temperatures. Pre-cooking in the microwave reduces those substances by as much as 90 percent.

You can also cut about half the fat out of the ground beef you use for spaghetti, chili, or other recipes that call for crumbled meat. It's easy:

- Brown the meat in a skillet.

- Place the meat on paper towels and blot it.

- Put the meat in a colander and rinse with hot water.

- Drain well.

Low fat doesn't necessarily mean low calorie

Watch out for the sugar content in many "low-fat" or "reduced-fat" foods. You may be cutting the fat but still getting a hefty dose of calories. And if one of your goals is to lose weight, you'll need to count calories. You can't drop pounds unless you burn more calories than you consume. That means eat less and exercise more.

Follow these suggestions for successful fat-free eating:

- Don't eat more. Just because you're choosing fat-free items doesn't mean you can empty the box. Eat the same amount you would eat of a regular product. And don't think that since you ate a fat-free cookie you can dish up a bowl of ice cream to go with it. Use low-fat items instead of, not in addition to, regular food.

- Stick with the basics. Make fresh fruits and vegetables, whole grains, beans, and lean meat the basis of your meal planning. These still guarantee whole-food nutrition with lots of vitamins, minerals, and fiber thrown in. Make fat-free items a special, small treat.

- Read your labels. Look out for high sugar and sodium content in fat-free foods. Many manufacturers add salt or sugar to make up for the lost taste of fat.

Read a food label like a pro

Do you spend hours in the grocery store trying to decipher food labels? You want to buy healthy, low-fat foods for your family, but sometimes you need an interpreter to explain the meanings behind those confusing numbers.

That's often the way food manufacturers want you to feel, especially if their product isn't quite as healthy as their advertising suggests. So arm yourself with a few basic terms, and you'll never again be at the mercy of food label fast talk.

Percent daily value. The most important number on a food label, percent daily value, is based on a 2,000-calorie-a-day diet. If you're watching your weight, you may not take in this many calories. But, you can still use the percent daily value to give you an idea of how a particular food fits into your nutritional plan. You should try to eat 100 percent of the daily value for each nutrient every day. If the listed percent daily value is 5 percent or less, you won't be getting much of that particular nutrient.

Nutrient claims. The government has established definitions for terms used on food labels.

- **High-protein**: at least 10 grams of high-quality protein per serving.

- **Fat-free:** less than 0.5 grams of fat per serving.

- **Low-fat:** 3 grams or less of fat per serving.

- **Good source of calcium**: at least 100 milligrams (mg) per serving.

- **Sugar-free:** less than 0.5 grams per serving.

- **Reduced or fewer calories**: at least 25 percent fewer calories per serving than the regular food.

- **Light:** one-third fewer calories or half the fat of the regular food, or a "low-calorie," "low-fat" food with half the sodium content of the regular food.

- **Low-sodium**: no more than 140 mg of sodium per serving.

- **Lightly salted**: at least 50 percent less sodium per serving than the regular form.

- **Reduced**: at least 25 percent less fat, sodium, or calories than the regular version.

American Heart Association symbol. If all the numbers still confuse you, there's another way to quickly pick out heart-healthy foods. Just look for the American Heart Association symbol, a heart with a check-mark in it. This means that particular food has met a specific set of AHA guidelines, including the Food and Drug Administration and U.S. Department of Agriculture government requirements for claims of fighting heart disease.

Without even reading a label, you'll know these products are low in saturated fat, sodium, and cholesterol, and they contain at least 10 percent of one or more of the following nutrients: protein, vitamin A, vitamin C, calcium, iron, or fiber. This makes it easy to buy foods that contribute to your family's health. Look for the AHA symbol on many of your favorites, like Cheerios.

If a certain product doesn't carry this symbol, however, don't dismiss it as unhealthy. Many manufacturers of heart-smart foods choose not to participate in the AHA Food Certification Program.

🐜 🐜 🐜
Frightening fat facts

Even if you're healthy and don't have high cholesterol, eating just one high-fat meal can keep your arteries from functioning properly for up to four hours.

You don't even have to swallow fat to experience its bad effects. Just by tasting it your triglyceride levels can go up, which means your blood clots more easily.

If you love pizza, watch out. Some pizza crusts alone contain around 28 percent trans fatty acids. These fatty acids, formed when vegetable oils are hardened by hydrogenation, are almost as bad for your heart as saturated fat.

Between the ages of 45 and 64, a woman's cholesterol level rises an average of 18 points. This is when you need to watch your fat intake like never before.

Beef and Vegetable Stir-fry

3/4 pound (12 ounces) boneless beef round steak
1 teaspoon olive oil
1/2 cup sliced carrots
1/2 cup sliced onion
1 tablespoon low-sodium soy sauce
1/8 teaspoon garlic powder
dash pepper
2 cups zucchini squash, cut in thin strips
1 tablespoon cornstarch
1/4 cup water

Trim all fat from steak. Slice steak across the grain into thin strips about 1/8 inch wide and 3 inches long. (Partially frozen meat is easier to slice).

Heat oil in frypan. Add beef strips and stir-fry over high heat, turning pieces constantly, until beef is no longer red (about 3 to 4 minutes).

Reduce heat. Add carrots, celery, onion, and seasonings. Cover and cook until carrots are slightly tender (3 to 5 minutes).

Add squash; cook until vegetables are tender-crisp (3 to 4 minutes).

Mix cornstarch and water until smooth; add slowly to beef mixture, stirring constantly. Cook until thickened and vegetables are coated with a thin glaze.

Makes 4 servings

Per serving: 200 Calories; 12g Fat (4g from saturated fat) (52% calories from fat); 18g Protein; 6g Carbohydrate; 50mg Cholesterol; 244mg Sodium

This is an official 5 A Day Recipe. This recipe is provided by the National Institutes of Health. Here's a way to still enjoy beef but limit some of the fat — add plenty of vegetables to the dish.

Ranch Potato Salad

3 medium russet potatoes, peeled and cubed
1/4 cup low-fat mayonnaise
1/2 cup fat-free ranch salad dressing
3/4 cup diced celery
1/2 cup thawed frozen peas
1 teaspoon paprika
1/4 cup chopped scallions
salt and freshly ground pepper to taste

Boil the potatoes for 10 to 15 minutes until done. Drain and set aside. Combine the remaining ingredients and toss well with the potatoes. Refrigerate for 1 hour before serving.

Makes 6 servings

Per serving: 110 Calories; 3g Fat (less than 1g from saturated fat)
(29% calories from fat); 2g Protein; 17g Carbohydrate; 0mg
Cholesterol; 315mg Sodium

American Diabetes website: www.diabetes.org
Book ordering number 1-800-232-6733.

Reprinted with permission of the American Diabetes Association, from
Flavorful Seasons Cookbook, by K. Spicer. ©1996.

Ranch-Style Vegetables

1 cup cauliflower, broken into bite-sized pieces
2 cups broccoli, broken into bite-sized pieces
3/4 cup sliced carrots
1/2 cup sliced celery
1/2 cup chopped onion
1/4 teaspoon dried dill weed
1 1/2 tablespoons lemon juice
2 tablespoons nonfat or reduced-fat ranch-style dressing

Fill a 1 1/2 quart microwave-safe dish with vegetables. Add
dill and lemon juice. Cover and microwave 5 to 8 minutes,
stirring every two minutes.

Drain, mix in dressing, and serve.

Makes 4 servings

Per serving: 47 Calories; less than 1g Fat (5.1% calories from fat);
2g Protein; 10g Carbohydrate; 0mg Cholesterol; 189mg Sodium

This is an official 5 A Day Recipe. This recipe is provided by the
National Institutes of Health. You can use any combination of fresh vegetables
you have available. This recipe provides each person served with more than
two servings of vegetables.

Magnesium

Amazing mineral is vital for heart health

Magnesium is probably just another entry in the periodic table you memorized briefly and then forgot about back in high school chemistry. Don't worry — you don't need to know its chemical symbol, but you should know what this amazing mineral can do for your health. It's been called a major discovery in natural healing, especially in matters of the heart. One study of over 15,000 people found that magnesium levels are strongly related to blood pressure, cholesterol levels, heart disease, diabetes, and atherosclerosis.

Many people think they get enough magnesium through their diet — after all the recommended dietary allowance (RDA) for adults over age 30 is only 420 milligrams (mg) for men and 320 mg for women. But, in reality, most people get about 200 mg a day.

Whole, natural, and unrefined foods are the best sources of magnesium, but the typical diet just doesn't contain enough of these. Most of the foods you eat are peeled, freeze-dried, bleached, preserved, refined, flavored, or filtered. The magnesium, and most other nutrients, have been processed right out of them.

So how do you know if you have a magnesium deficiency? It may take a special blood test to find out for sure, but if you experience weakness, confusion, fatigue, muscle cramps, insomnia, loss of appetite, stress, irritability, or heart disturbances, bring the matter up with your doctor.

There are many reasons why you could have low levels of magnesium — if you don't get enough of this important mineral in your diet, if you've depleted your body's stores through persistent vomiting or diarrhea, if you suffer from an intestinal disease, or if you are an alcoholic. Certain drugs used to treat heart failure, especially diuretics and digitalis, can cause a magnesium deficiency, too.

If you fall into any of these categories, talk with your doctor. He'll probably suggest eating more magnesium-rich foods, taking oral supplements, or both.

6 ways magnesium can heal your heart

Magnesium is a critically important mineral for your heart. Here's how it helps.

Controls cholesterol. If you are currently being treated for high cholesterol, you may want to consider adding magnesium supplements to your daily regimen. Studies have shown that magnesium can make certain cholesterol-lowering drugs, like Pravastatin, more effective. The result — even lower LDL cholesterol.

Noninsulin-dependent diabetes sometimes goes hand-in-hand with high cholesterol. If this is your situation, magnesium should be in your medicine cabinet. It could greatly improve your cholesterol levels.

Balances blood pressure. Magnesium helps to control blood pressure in three ways. First, it keeps nerve fibers from releasing epinephrine, a hormone that constricts your blood vessels. Relaxed blood vessels mean more room for your blood to flow and that means lower blood pressure.

Second, it balances the amount of sodium and potassium in your blood cells — less sodium, more potassium. When magnesium was given to a group of people with high blood pressure, researchers noticed that the sodium levels in their blood decreased and their blood pressure came down. The higher the magnesium levels, the lower their blood pressure.

And last, magnesium interacts with another very important mineral, calcium, in a special way. These two are sometimes thought of as opposites, since calcium contracts muscles and magnesium relaxes them. Because of the way they interact, magnesium has sometimes been called a natural calcium channel-blocker. It keeps calcium from entering the cells in your arteries and heart muscles and constricting them. Relaxed arteries and muscles are important if you suffer from angina, high blood pressure, or congestive heart failure.

Regulates heart rhythm. Magnesium helps your muscles relax after a contraction, a process especially important for normal heart rhythm. A magnesium deficiency seems to increase the risk of sudden death in people who have heart failure.

Takes aim at atherosclerosis. Scientists think too little magnesium in your body may be the missing connection between simply having heart disease risk factors and actually developing heart disease, like atherosclerosis. Not enough magnesium can cause a chain reaction of trouble within your cells and blood vessels that results in narrowed or inflamed arteries, blood clots, and a buildup of cholesterol in your bloodstream.

Improves survival odds. People who die from heart attacks have less magnesium in their heart cells than people who die from other causes. This discovery led researchers to try using magnesium to prevent and treat heart attacks. They observed several benefits — the heart attacks were generally less severe, and fewer people died after suffering a heart attack.

It seems that magnesium helps in several ways.

- It steadies your heart rate and helps prevent an irregular heartbeat.

- It keeps blood cells from clumping together and forming clots.

- It relaxes and enlarges your arteries, which improves blood and oxygen flow to your heart.

- It stimulates the production of energy, which keeps your heart pumping.

Revives your valves. The chambers in your heart contract and relax in a regular rhythm known as your heartbeat. The valves between these chambers open and close in sync with your heartbeat to allow your blood to keep flowing through. When a valve is slightly deformed or becomes injured through inflammation, infection, or simply age, part of the tissue collapses into the heart chamber, and the valve doesn't close as tightly as it should. Blood leaks from one chamber to another, causing shortness of breath, fatigue, and sometimes chest pain or a heart murmur.

Mitral valve prolapse (MVP), a common condition affecting the mitral valve, seems to be associated with low levels of magnesium. A recent study showed that giving magnesium supplements to people who have MVP greatly improved their symptoms, including chest pain, anxiety, palpitations, weakness, and shortness of breath.

The best way to boost your magnesium

You don't always have to take a pill. Simply getting a little extra magnesium from the foods you eat can make a big difference in your cholesterol levels. Foods like seafood, dark green vegetables, and even chocolate can boost your magnesium and give you added ammunition in your fight against high cholesterol and other heart-related problems. Here are some other choices:

green leafy vegetables	nuts	peas	beans
whole cereal grains	tofu	seeds	bananas
dried fruits	berries	currants	dates
canned pineapple	citrus	papaya	avocado

If you have too much fat in your diet, your body may not be absorbing magnesium very well. That's just one more reason to cut back on the fat.

Another thing to consider is your drinking water. Since it's been proven that people with high levels of magnesium in their drinking water are less likely to suffer from heart failure, some experts want to explore the possibility of adding extra magnesium to everyday sources, like table salt and the water supply. Changes like these are easier on the general population, since it doesn't mean remembering to take a pill or buying anything special.

Hard water is generally high in minerals and actually contains more magnesium than soft water. If your home has a water softener, you may want to consider magnesium supplements.

Beware of the dangers of too much magnesium

Moderation is the magic word when it comes to magnesium. That's because too much can make you very sick, causing nausea, vomiting, or even paralysis and death.

If you regularly consume large amounts of over-the-counter antacids, laxatives, or pain relievers that contain magnesium, you may be poisoning yourself. One woman who had been taking two bottles of magnesium-containing antacids a day for several months learned that lesson the hard way. She ended up paralyzed, in a hospital on life support, before routine blood work uncovered her massive magnesium overload.

She was one of the lucky ones. According to a study from the Food and Drug Administration, 14 people have died and several others have been hospitalized or disabled from magnesium poisonings since 1968.

Older people are particularly prone to magnesium poisoning because they often have indigestion and constipation and frequently turn to over-the-counter remedies for relief. In addition, many people think if a little works well, a lot works better, so they take far more than recommended. Problems also arise because older people's kidneys don't work as well as they used to, and they don't remove excess magnesium from the body as well as they should.

If you have a stomach or intestinal disorder and take several drugs, especially narcotics or anticholinergics (drugs used to block impulses from the central nervous system, including some antidepressants, antihistamines, antiparkinsonism drugs, and muscles relaxers), you have an especially high risk of experiencing side effects from a magnesium overdose.

Signs of a magnesium overdose include lightheadedness, low blood pressure, muscle weakness, confusion, heart rhythm abnormalities, nausea, and vomiting. If you have any of these symptoms, stop taking the magnesium supplements and see your doctor immediately.

To protect yourself, carefully read all labels on any over-the-counter medicines you take. If possible, substitute a product that contains magnesium for another product that doesn't. Never take a higher dosage than the manufacturer recommends. In addition, don't take antacids and laxatives at the same time. Let your doctor know about any over-the-counter medicine you use regularly.

And finally, if you have kidney or heart disease, don't take magnesium supplements without your doctor's approval.

Oven Wedge Fries

2 potatoes, large sized
1 teaspoon olive oil

Seasoning suggestions:

2 cloves garlic, finely chopped
Italian seasoning spice mix
chili powder
paprika
cayenne red pepper

Preheat oven to 400 degrees F.

Cut potatoes into quarters. Then cut each quarter into wedges with the wedge part (area with the skin) about 1/2 to 1/3 inch wide. Coat Teflon cookie sheet with 1 teaspoon oil. Lay wedges on the cookie sheet, one side down.

Place cookie sheet on the oven rack about 7 inches from the oven bottom. Bake for 7 minutes (or until the bottom and edges start browning), then flip wedges over to their other side and sprinkle any seasonings over the top.

Bake for another 7 minutes, or until the wedges are nicely brown and cooked thoroughly.

Makes 4 servings

Per serving: 45 Calories; 1g Fat (less than 1g from saturated fat) (23% calories from fat); 1g Protein; 8g Carbohydrate; 0mg Cholesterol; 3mg Sodium

This is an official 5 A Day Recipe. This recipe provided by the Idaho Potato Commission.

Spinach Ricotta Dumplings with Marinara Sauce

10 ounces chopped frozen spinach, thawed and squeezed dry
15 ounces part-skim ricotta cheese
1 cup bread crumbs
1/2 cup egg substitute
1/4 cup grated Parmesan cheese
2 cloves garlic, crushed
1/2 teaspoon ground nutmeg
1/4 cup flour
28 ounces marinara sauce, garden-style

Combine spinach, ricotta, bread crumbs, egg substitute, Parmesan, garlic, and nutmeg. Form into balls about the size of golf balls. Roll lightly in flour. Chill at least 2 hours.

Heat marinara sauce. Cook half of dumplings in a large pot of boiling salted water. They will sink and then float to surface when cooked (about 6 minutes). Remove dumplings with a slotted spoon. Repeat with remaining dumplings.

Divide dumplings among six dishes. Top each with sauce.

Makes 6 servings

Per serving: 341 Calories; 14g Fat (5g from saturated fat) (36% calories from fat); 19g Protein; 38g Carbohydrate; 25mg Cholesterol; 1183mg Sodium

Reprinted with permission from The Art of Cooking for the Diabetic by Mary Abbott Hess, 1996

Movement Therapy

Recharge your 'battery' with ancient therapies

Moving your body is good for your heart, but if you're just not a jump-around-in-a-leotard-and-sweat kind of person, here's good news. You don't have to do strenuous exercise to strengthen your heart. Other types of "movement therapies" have been shown to have a positive effect on heart health.

Tai chi (tie-chee). This ancient Chinese movement system consists of flowing, gentle movements performed very slowly. The slow motion allows you to breathe properly, concentrate, and relax.

Students of Tai chi learn different forms. A form is a sequence of movements that can take from five to 30 minutes to perform. People practicing Tai chi sometimes look as though they are moving slowly through water.

Tai chi is particularly well-suited to older people. Studies show it improves balance and helps prevent falls that can be disastrous to the elderly.

Researchers have also found that Tai chi can benefit your heart by helping to lower your blood pressure. One study at Johns Hopkins Medical Center found that Tai chi lowered blood pressure almost as much as moderate aerobics. People in the study who participated in Tai chi lowered their systolic blood pressure an average of 7 points, while the people who did aerobics lowered theirs by an average of 8.4 points. A study in Great Britain had similar results, with one exception. While aerobics and Tai chi both lowered systolic blood pressure, only the Tai chi lowered diastolic blood pressure, too.

Yoga. There are three aspects to yoga — exercise, breathing, and meditation. The exercise helps improve muscle tone, circulation, and flexibility. Learning to breathe properly and meditate helps relieve stress and improve concentration.

There are several different styles of yoga. Hatha yoga represents the physical kind of yoga and involves learning different postures, or "asanas." Ha means "sun," and tha means "moon."

Most studies on the health benefits of yoga have been done on Hatha yoga. In several studies, yoga reduced blood pressure and cholesterol levels. And, according to a recent study, people with congestive heart failure showed improvement when they practiced yoga-type breathing exercises.

If you decide to practice yoga, find a reputable instructor because doing the techniques improperly may result in injury. Here's something else you should keep in mind — yoga requires practice, but the rewards should be well worth your effort.

Nuts

Cracking the secret to better heart health

It may sound a bit nutty, but munching a handful of crunchy nuts may be the easiest way to protect your heart.

Nuts have been a diet staple for centuries. They are a good source of protein, fiber, and vitamins and minerals important to heart health, like folic acid, vitamin E, potassium, and magnesium.

Although nuts are high in fat, they are low in saturated fat and cholesterol free. Most nuts are a rich source of monounsaturated fatty acids, the same kind found in olive oil, or polyunsaturated fatty acids, which are also found in fish oil.

Researchers studying 30,000 Seventh Day Adventists found that those who ate nuts at least five times a week reduced their risk of heart attack by 50 percent, compared with those who ate them less than once a week.

Other studies have found that adding nuts to your diet can lower your cholesterol level. In one study, people who added almonds to their diets lowered their total cholesterol by 7 percent and their LDL cholesterol by 10 percent. People who added walnuts to their diets lowered their total cholesterol by 5 percent and their LDL cholesterol by 9 percent.

Before you get carried away and buy a hydraulic nutcracker, keep in mind that nuts are high in calories. An ounce of nuts usually has between 160 to 200 calories, which can add up quickly. If those extra calories cause you to gain weight, you may cancel out the health benefits of eating nuts.

Keep some nuts around for quick, nutritious snacking. Be daring and toss some in your oatmeal or cereal in the morning, or add a few to your bread dough, pancake or muffin batter, or fruit salad.

Many varieties of nuts contain a lot of added salt. If you're salt sensitive, check the label for sodium content.

Nut (1 oz)	Calories	Protein	Fiber	Folic acid	Potassium	Magnesium
English walnuts	182	4.05 g	1.36 g	19 mcg	143 mg	48 mg
Black walnuts	172	6.91 g	1.42 g	19 mcg	149 mg	57 mg
Peanuts	164	6.63 g	2.24 g	41 mcg	184 mg	49 mg
Pecans	189	2.20 g	2.15 g	11 mcg	111 mg	36 mg
Cashews	163	4.34 g	.85 g	20 mcg	160 mg	74 mg
Almonds	167	5.66 g	3.09 g	17 mcg	208 mg	84 mg
Pistachios	164	5.84 g	3.06 g	16 mcg	310 mg	45 mg

The nut that isn't a nut

One of the most popular and healthy nuts — the peanut — isn't really a nut at all. It's a legume, like beans and peas. Peanuts may also be called groundnuts, earth nuts, and, in the South, goobers. The plants grow above the ground, but after flowering, the branches bend downward and the pods become buried under the soil.

About half of the peanut crop every year is used to make peanut butter, a staple in most schoolchildren's lunch boxes.

Although peanuts aren't really nuts, they have the same nutritional benefits. They're high in protein, vitamins, and minerals, and they contain polyunsaturated fatty acids. Researchers say they also contain another substance that may help your heart — resveratrol. This antioxidant, also found in grape skins, is partly responsible for red wine's ability to lower heart disease risk. (See the *Grapes and red wine* chapter for more information.)

So now, instead of having a glass of wine with your dinner, just have a peanut butter and jelly sandwich instead. Cheers!

🐜 🐜

The latest news about nuts

Almonds. There are two varieties of almonds — sweet and bitter. The kind you're familiar with is probably sweet because bitter almonds are illegal in the United States. Raw bitter almonds contain prussic acid, which is toxic, but the heating process destroys the poison.

Pine nuts. These nuts are found inside the pine cones of several varieties of pine trees. The pine cones usually must be heated in order to remove the nuts. This process makes pine nuts rather expensive. They also have a high fat content, which causes them to turn rancid quickly. They can be stored in the refrigerator for up to three months, or frozen for up to nine months.

Pistachios. These pale green nuts come in a tan shell, although sometimes the shell is dyed red with a vegetable dye or blanched white. When buying unshelled pistachios, look for ones with shells that are partially open. Not only does it make cracking the hard shells easier, it means the nut inside is fully ripened.

Pecans. This member of the hickory family has the highest fat content of any nut — over 70 percent. They are probably most well-known for helping make Southern pecan pie so decadently rich and delicious. Like pine nuts, their high fat content invites rancidity. Store shelled pecans in the refrigerator for up to three months, or the freezer for up to six months.

Macadamia nuts. The macadamia tree was first grown in Australia and was named after John McAdam, the man who first cultivated it. Hawaii is now the largest exporter of macadamias. Their exotic, sweet taste compliment many different kinds of dishes.

Cashews. This buttery-tasting nut has a shell that is very toxic, so great care is taken in shelling and cleaning them. They contain about 48 percent fat.

Walnuts. Because the wrinkled shell of this nut resembled the brain, ancient doctors used them to treat head ailments. Today, adding them to your cooking may not help your head, but it could head off heart disease.

Strawberry Yogurt Breakfast Split

1 banana
4 ounces (1 cup) fresh strawberries
4 ounces (1/2 cup) vanilla yogurt
1 tablespoon chopped, toasted almonds

Peel and split 1 banana. Place banana halves in serving bowl.

Top with strawberries, yogurt, and almonds.

Makes 1 serving

Per serving: 191 Calories; 6g Fat (3g from saturated fat) (28% calories from fat); 6g Protein; 31g Carbohydrate; 14mg Cholesterol; 55mg Sodium

This is an official 5 A Day Recipe. This recipe is provided by the California Strawberry Advisory Board.

Waldorf Salad

Tart apples include Rome, Jonathan, and Granny Smith varieties.

3 medium (1 pound) tart apples
2/3 cup thinly sliced celery
1/2 cup walnuts, halves and pieces
1/3 cup light or reduced-fat mayonnaise
1/3 cup unsweetened applesauce
2 teaspoons lemon juice
1/4 teaspoon salt
1/4 teaspoon freshly ground pepper
6 crisp lettuce leaves

Wash and core apples. Cut them into bite-sized slices with peel on them. Put apples in a large bowl; add celery and walnuts.

To make the dressing, mix remaining ingredients in a small bowl. Gently toss apple mixture with dressing. Serve on lettuce leaves.

Makes 6 servings

Per serving: 122 Calories; 8g Fat (1g from saturated fat) (53% calories from fat); 1g Protein; 14g Carbohydrate; 0mg Cholesterol; 144mg Sodium

Reprinted with permission from The Art of Cooking for the Diabetic by Mary Abbott Hess, 1996

Potassium

Conquer high blood pressure with vital mineral

Wouldn't you rather eat delicious fresh fruits and vegetables to help keep your blood pressure under control than take a pill every day? Researchers have proven that foods high in potassium, like many fruits and vegetables, can help lower your blood pressure.

In one study, people took their high blood pressure medicine as usual, but they also ate foods rich in potassium. By the end of the study, most of them were able to reduce their medication by more than 50 percent and still keep their blood pressure down. Numerous other studies have also found that an adequate potassium intake helps keep your blood pressure under control and lowers your risk of heart and artery disease and stroke.

Potassium may be particularly helpful in reducing the effects of a high-salt diet. Several studies suggest that people with a low potassium intake are more likely to be salt sensitive. This means eating salt causes their blood pressure to rise. However, when those people increased their intake of potassium-rich foods, their salt sensitivity decreased.

Some researchers think primitive societies avoid high blood pressure, not because of their low sodium intake, but because of their high potassium intake. Those societies don't have access to sodium-laden processed foods that developed countries do. They rely more on fresh fruits and vegetables, which are high in potassium.

Why is this mineral so important to your heart? Potassium is an electrolyte that is essential to electrical reactions in your body, including your heart. It also helps keep your heartbeat steady by helping your muscles contract, and it assists your kidneys in removing waste from your body.

There is no recommended dietary allowance (RDA) for potassium. The estimated minimum requirement for adults is 2,000 milligrams (mg) a day. Although most people don't get enough potassium, a true deficiency, which causes you to become sick, is unusual in healthy people. Diarrhea, vomiting, kidney disease, fasting, and the use of diuretics or laxatives can also cause you to become deficient in potassium.

Do your heart and your taste buds a favor and include plenty of potassium-rich foods in your diet.

Food	Serving size	Potassium (mg)
Apricots, dried	1 cup	1,791
Avocado, Florida	1 medium	1,484
Figs, dried	1 cup	1,416
Prunes, dried	1 cup	1,199
Acorn squash, baked	1 cup	895
Kidney beans, canned	1 cup	658
Potato, baked	1 medium	610
Cantaloupe, cubed	1 cup	494
Banana	1 medium	451
Tomato juice	1/2 cup	268
Guava	1 medium	256
Orange	1 medium	255
Peach	1 medium	171

Food or supplement — Which one is best?

It's very unlikely you would get too much potassium from your diet, but beware of supplements. If you're thinking about taking a potassium supplement, check with your doctor first. Too much potassium can be more dangerous than too little. Potassium overdose can cause nausea, diarrhea, weakness, paralysis, kidney damage, irregular heartbeat, and even death.

If you're taking a diuretic for high blood pressure, your doctor might recommend a potassium supplement because diuretics can cause you to lose potassium. However, if you're taking a potassium-sparing diuretic as well as a potassium supplement, you could be getting too much.

Other medications that might contribute to a buildup of potassium include ACE inhibitors, beta-blockers, heparin, and nonsteroidal anti-inflammatory drugs (NSAIDs), like aspirin and ibuprofen.

Some disorders, like kidney disease and Addison's disease, make you more likely to accumulate excess amounts of potassium in your body. And people who have diabetes may have a defect in the kidney's ability to regulate levels of potassium. If you have one of these disorders, you have to be particularly careful about your potassium intake.

Although salt substitutes can help you cut down on your sodium, and maybe lower your blood pressure, be aware that many of them contain potassium. If you're taking supplements and using a potassium-containing salt substitute, you might end up with dangerously high levels of potassium.

Grand Slam Dinner

Make this speedy dish even faster by picking up pre-shredded cabbage and carrots at your grocery store's salad bar or in ready-to-use packages.

2 teaspoons sugar
1/2 teaspoon salt
1 teaspoon pepper
3/4 cup red wine vinegar
2 tablespoons olive oil
1/2 teaspoon cumin
4 lean pork center loin chops
1 medium onion, chopped
8 red potatoes, quartered
1/2 cup sliced red cabbage
2 cups sliced green cabbage
3/4 cup shredded carrot
1 green apple, chopped

Mix the first five ingredients to make a dressing. Pour about one-fourth of the mixture into a shallow bowl; reserve the rest for the cabbage salad.

Dip the pork chops into the shallow bowl of dressing, turning to coat, and then sprinkle each chop with cumin. Place pork chops in a metal baking pan, cover with onion, and pour dressing used to dip the pork chops over the top.

Broil for about 7 minutes, turn, and broil for 6 minutes more.

Meanwhile, microwave potato quarters for 5 to 7 minutes, then place them under the broiler as the pork chops are being turned.

Slice and shred salad ingredients and toss them with remaining three-fourths of the dressing in a large bowl. Serve pork and potatoes along with salad.

Makes 4 servings

Per serving: 484 Calories; 22g Fat (6g from saturated fat) (39% calories from fat); 27g Protein; 48g Carbohydrate; 75mg Cholesterol; 502mg Sodium

This is an official 5 A Day Recipe. This recipe is provided by the National Institutes of Health.

Layered Italian Salad with Basil Vinaigrette

This recipe provides each person served with about two servings of vegetables.

4 Roma tomatoes, thinly sliced
1 green zucchini, thinly sliced
2 yellow zucchini, thinly sliced
salt and pepper to taste

Basil Vinaigrette or Nonfat Basil Vinegar:

1/2 cup balsamic vinegar
1/2 tablespoon olive oil (optional)
8 fresh basil leaves, finely chopped (or 2 teaspoons dried basil)

On a serving plate, layer alternate slices of tomato, yellow zucchini, and green zucchini in a stairway pattern so all vegetables show.

Mix dressing ingredients and add to vegetables. Add salt and pepper to taste.

Makes 4 servings

Per serving: 56 Calories; 2g Fat (less than 1g from saturated fat) (30% calories from fat); 2g Protein; 10g Carbohydrate; 0mg Cholesterol; 13mg Sodium

This is an official 5 A Day Recipe. This recipe is provided by the National Institutes of Health.

Prunes

A prune by any name would taste as healthy

Movie stars frequently change their ordinary, given names to something more glamorous once they're in the spotlight. That's happened with your old friend the prune.

Ever since researchers discovered that prunes are packed with antioxidants, this dried fruit has gotten lots of attention. Who knew so much goodness was hiding inside that black, wrinkly package?

Like the star it hopes to become, the prune has changed its name and is now known as a "dried plum." The Food and Drug Administration approved the change, which was recommended by the California Prune Board. It hopes to shed the prune's image of a food for the elderly and target it to the young and health conscious. Market surveys show the name change is a winner, and this new celebrity should appear soon at a grocery near you.

Prunes give you lots of fiber, protect you from free radical damage, and maybe even lower your cholesterol. They are also a good source of potassium — important for a healthy heart and strong bones. And you can eat 10 sweet, chewy dried plums filled with nutrition for only 200 calories. Not bad for a food that was rescued from hospital and nursing home cafeterias.

Dried plums knock down high cholesterol

Eating a diet high in fiber can help lower your cholesterol, and a study of prunes helped prove it.

Researchers in the Department of Nutrition at the University of California, Davis, gave a group of 41 men with mildly high cholesterol 12 prunes each day for four weeks. They then gave the same men a couple of glasses of grape juice daily for four more weeks. The men were told not to change their eating or exercise habits during the study.

Tests showed that LDL cholesterol — the kind you want to keep low — was significantly lower during the prune period than during the grape juice period. This is great news if your cholesterol is starting to creep upwards and you don't want to take medicine. Lower cholesterol means you're less likely to develop heart disease.

Get antioxidant protection

For years, scientists have wondered what people can do to hold on to the health and vitality of their youth. The latest thinking is that antioxidants — free radical fighters found mainly in fruits and vegetables — are the key to keeping young and avoiding cell damage.

Researchers have measured and studied antioxidants in food at the Jean Mayer USDA Human Nutrition Research Center on Aging at Tufts University in Boston. Of all the foods tested, the prune had the highest Oxygen Radical Absorbance Capacity (ORAC) score. At 5,770 ORACs per 3 1/2-ounce serving, it registered more than twice as many antioxidants as the next highest food — its wrinkled cousin, the raisin.

Scientists think antioxidants may be an important key to protecting yourself from diseases of aging and even cancer. In fact, the loss of brain function in certain diseases like Parkinson's and Alzheimer's seems to be from free radical damage. If these high antioxidant foods can protect you from free radicals, imagine all the sickness you might avoid.

The USDA's Agricultural Research Service Administrator Floyd P. Horn has seen the future of treating age-related diseases, and it looks a lot like your grandma's vegetable garden.

"If these findings are borne out in further research," he says, "young and middle-aged people may be able to reduce risk of diseases of aging — including senility — simply by adding high-ORAC foods to their diets."

By studying blood samples from different groups of people, the researchers concluded that you can raise the levels of antioxidants in your blood by eating more fruits and vegetables. For now, they're recommending you eat enough fruits and vegetables to total between 3,000 and 5,000 ORAC units of antioxidants daily. Since most of the foods tested scored in the hundreds, you'd have to eat many servings to reach 3,000.

But chew on this: eating just seven prunes a day can put you well over the 3,000 mark. All the other fruits and vegetables you eat would be gravy. Make sure you eat a variety, though, because each fruit and vegetable has different protective nutrients.

🐚 🐚 🐚

Prunes can replace fat

You can use prunes to make a puree substitution for oil or butter in recipes.

Just puree about 1 1/3 cups of pitted prunes with 6 tablespoons of hot water. This should make about a cup of prune puree that will keep in the refrigerator for up to one month. Use half the recommended fat in a recipe, then add half that amount of pureed prunes.

For example, if a recipe calls for a cup of oil or butter, use 1/2 cup of oil, then add 1/4 cup of prune puree. You can use this puree in cakes, muffins, cookies — even brownies.

🐚 🐚

Relaxation

Learn to use your mind to help your heart

You may think meditation is some kind of unusual, far-out Eastern religious practice, but meditation can also be used as a focus in Christian Bible study or prayer. Over the last 20 years, research shows all kinds of people have been enjoying its benefits.

A study of older meditators, average age 81 years, found improvements in learning, speaking, and thinking. Their mental health was better, and they felt more in control of their lives. After three years, their survival rate was about 94 percent, much higher than the nonmeditators in the study.

Researchers also claim meditating keeps you out of the doctor's office. According to insurance statistics, meditators require 30 to 87 percent less medical attention than nonmeditators, which saves lots of time and money. It helps relieve chronic pain, anxiety, and substance abuse and can be especially helpful in preventing and treating heart disease.

Side step artery damage. Every time you feel extreme stress, your blood pressure goes up. Researchers say extreme increases in blood pressure can damage artery walls. This increases your risk of cholesterol deposits forming within your arteries. And that, of course, means atherosclerosis, heart attacks, and strokes. To protect your arteries, you must learn to deal with the stress in your life.

If you're still not convinced, think about this. When lipids, which are fats like cholesterol, join with oxygen, they damage your artery walls and start the process that ends in atherosclerosis. But in one study, people practicing a specific type of meditation had 15 percent less of this oxidized lipid in their blood. Researchers think lowering stress with meditation is a natural way to lower your risk of heart disease.

Dodge high blood pressure. What a difference relaxing can make. Even if you have all the risk factors for developing high blood pressure, meditation can help bring it down. In fact, if you meditate regularly, you can control your pressure even under pressure. That's great news if you're looking for a way to take charge of your own health. In a study at the University of California at Los Angeles School of Medicine, people with high blood pressure learned how to relax, manage their stress, and cut out negative thinking. As a result, more than half of them were able to go completely without their blood pressure medicine, even a year later.

Steer clear of disease. Physical stress is known to suppress your immune system, leaving your body more open to damage and disease. Regular meditation counteracts the stress, allowing your immune system to function normally.

Focus on an active life. If you want to improve your quality of life despite a heart condition, consider meditation. When a small group of people with known heart disease began practicing meditation, they were able to exercise longer and harder, and their heart rate and blood pressure stayed lower than those who exercised but did not meditate.

🐜 🐜 🐜

Talking may be hazardous to your health

Talking too much may irritate your friends, but did you know it could also be a health hazard? Studies by Dr. James Lynch of the University of Maryland Medical School show that listening, rather than talking, lowers blood pressure. According to reports, 98 percent of the 178 people studied had their blood pressures surge when they started talking.

The highs and lows of blood pressure levels won't hurt people with normal blood pressure, Dr. Lynch explains, but in someone with high blood pressure, the highs can be dangerous.

Many people with high blood pressure do not speak calmly, which causes their blood pressures to rise even further. Dr. Lynch claims that the louder and faster a person talks, the higher his blood pressure. People who emphasize their words, talk "breathlessly," use hand motions, interrupt, or talk over someone else seem to experience the highest rise in blood pressure.

Dr. Lynch believes that slower speaking, combined with breathing more deeply and regularly during speech, helps to lower blood pressure. Anyone with speech-induced blood pressure problems can learn to speak more slowly, he says.

Learning to listen and focusing on what the other person is saying might lower stress and reduce the load on the heart. Most people with chronic high blood pressure do not really "listen" to a conversation, Lynch explains. These people are so worried about how they will reply that they are defensive even when they are listening, and their blood pressure doesn't drop as much as it does in a person who truly listens.

The next time you visit your friends or family, listen to what they have to say. Your blood pressure will thank you for it.

🐜 🐜

Simple technique melts away stress

Relaxing your body makes you feel good, but if you are at risk of a heart attack, serious relaxation training is vital. Learning how to relax is more than just a physical exercise, more than spending an hour in a bubble bath. You must loosen tensed muscles and allow screaming nerves to quiet down, but more importantly, you have to let emotional stress go. Several chapters in this book discuss different ways to do this: the *Alexander technique*, *Anger arresters*, *Job-stress solutions*, and *Aromatherapy*, just to name a few. The kind of relaxation discussed here is closer to meditation than anything else.

You can learn the technique of relaxing without a teacher if you are patient and really practice. Devoting 20 minutes twice a day while learning is ideal. Most people find that setting a particular time and place helps them get into the relaxation habit and stick to it.

This progressive relaxation technique is good to master before moving on to any other type of meditation. It is a powerful, yet simple, process. You can practice it lying down or sitting up. Here's how:

- Choose a quiet, comfortable spot.

- Take a few extra-deep, slow breaths.

- Close your eyes and progressively relax your body one muscle group at a time. Start by clenching the muscles of your toes to tighten them while you count to 10. Then relax them for a count of 10. Do the same with the muscles of your feet.

- Continue up your body, tensing and relaxing each muscle group. By the time you reach the top of your head, all the tension in your body should just melt away.

Studies have shown if you combine normal rehabilitation after a heart attack with relaxation therapy, your chances of suffering another heart attack, needing heart surgery, or dying from a heart-related incident are much lower. In fact, just by learning and practicing this simple technique, hospitalizations for heart problems can be reduced by more than 30 percent.

Decoding your body language

You may think you have life's stresses under control, but are you sure? Your body may be saying something different. Quick — stop what you're doing and take this quiz to see just how relaxed you are. You're in good shape if you have:

- dry palms
- loose jaw
- dropped shoulders
- slow, abdominal breathing
- warm hands
- smooth forehead muscles
- slow heartbeat

Now think about your daily routine. You can count yourself among the truly unruffled if you have:

- deep, restful sleep
- few headaches
- no regular muscle pain
- normal bowels

If you had to unclench your jaw or loosen your shoulders while you were reading this, you've got some unconscious stress going on. For your health's sake, learn how to make relaxation a conscious part of your life.

Relax your way to health

In the 1970s, there was a lot of concern about the effects of stress on the heart. That's why Dr. Herbert Benson and his associates at Harvard University decided to study the claims of people who were practicing meditation. They found that, indeed, their blood pressure, heartbeat, and respiration did slow down. In fact, they discovered everything that increased with stress, decreased during meditation.

Since what they found was the exact opposite of the stress response, Benson called these changes "the relaxation response." Based on this research, he developed a simple meditation almost anyone could do.

He wanted it to be acceptable to all people, regardless of their religious beliefs, so he suggested you choose a word or expression that has a special meaning to you. You might use a word that reflects the feeling you want, like "peace" or "joy." Or you might repeat a prayer or verse of scripture.

To practice the relaxation response, get in a comfortable position, close your eyes, breathe deeply, relax your muscles, and let your stress melt away.

Rhubarb

Lower cholesterol with fiber-rich rhubarb

If you're lucky, your grandmother had a special family rhubarb pie recipe. If not, start your own tradition and add this sweet and tart winter vegetable to your regular menu.

As far as healthy eating goes, it's hard to beat rhubarb. It's full of potassium, calcium, vitamin A, and vitamin C. It's also a great source of fiber, and it's as good for your heart as guar gum or psyllium. That's because it lowers bad LDL cholesterol without affecting your good HDL cholesterol.

Rhubarb looks like colorful celery, but its sharp flavor is nothing at all like celery's. In fact, most rhubarb recipes need a considerable amount of sugar just to tone down the intensity.

Choose crisp, brightly colored stalks for best flavor, but be sure to remove all the leaves before cooking. The leaves contain oxalic acid, which can be toxic.

Stewed Rhubarb

You may use fresh or frozen rhubarb for this recipe.

1 pound (4 cups) fresh or frozen rhubarb, diced
1/4 cup water
6 tablespoons sugar or the equivalent in artificial sweetener

Place diced rhubarb and water in a deep saucepan. Cover and bring to a boil. Reduce heat; simmer gently until rhubarb is very tender, about 10 to 15 minutes, stirring occasionally.

Remove from heat, add sweetener, and mix well. The amount of sweetener required depends largely upon the acidity or "sour" taste of the rhubarb you use. Taste and adjust the amount of sweetener accordingly.

Serve warm or chilled.

Frozen unsweetened rhubarb is sold in 1-pound packages. The amount of fresh rhubarb to pick or buy, in order to end up with the same quantity — 4 cups uncooked — depends upon how much top and bottom is left on before cleaning and cutting.

Makes 4 servings

Per serving: 25 Calories; less than 1g Fat (0g from saturated fat) (4% calories from fat); 1g Protein; 6g Carbohydrate; 0mg Cholesterol; 4mg Sodium

Reprinted with permission from The Art of Cooking for the Diabetic by Mary Abbott Hess, 1996

Salt

Should you shake your salt habit?

Salt's rock-solid reputation has gotten a bit shaky in the last few decades. It hasn't always been that way. For most of history, salt was a respected and valuable item. Roman soldiers were paid a "salarium," or salt money, which is the origin of the word salary. A good soldier was "worth his salt." And when Jesus said, "Ye are the salt of the earth," he meant it as a compliment.

Salt, also known as sodium chloride, is an important mineral that is 40 percent sodium and 60 percent chloride. You need a certain amount of salt to survive. A salty, mineral-rich fluid constantly bathes and nourishes the cells of your body.

Salt acts as an electrolyte. This means it helps regulate body fluids and helps maintain normal blood volume. It's also needed for the normal function of nerves and muscles.

The Food and Drug Administration recommends no more than 2,400 milligrams (mg) of sodium a day, but most people get 4,000 to 6,000 mg a day.

Your kidneys regulate the mineral and water balance in your body — about 98 percent of the salt you take in comes out in your urine. If you eat too much salt, your kidneys have to work harder, and you may wash out other important minerals, like calcium, along with the sodium. If you eat a lot of salt, you also need to increase your water intake.

About 60 percent of the people who have high blood pressure have kidneys that don't work very well. If your kidneys can't get rid of the excess salt you take in, and you have extra sodium, chloride, and water in your body, the compartments that hold the cell-bathing fluid have to expand. This could cause high blood pressure, swelling, and fluid in your lungs. Retaining fluid is a factor in congestive heart failure and kidney disease.

Does that mean eating salt will raise your blood pressure? Intersalt, a huge international study, found a link between sodium intake and high blood pressure. Usually, the more salt you eat, the more you excrete in your urine. Intersalt found that people with a high sodium content in their urine were more likely to have high blood pressure. The association was stronger for older people.

Other studies have found that not everyone responds to salt with an increase in blood pressure. The people who do are called salt-sensitive. These are the people who really need to watch their salt intake.

How do you know if you're salt-sensitive? Right now, the only way to be sure is to monitor your blood pressure and salt intake carefully over a period of time to see if eating salt raises your blood pressure. This can be a very time-consuming process.

Because of the few studies that indicate low salt may be bad for you, some researchers think a blanket recommendation of the same salt intake level for everyone isn't a good idea.

If you have high blood pressure, most studies indicate that limiting your salt intake will help lower it. If you don't have high blood pressure, you don't have to be as careful about salt, but it's probably still a good idea not to overdo it.

&. &. &.

Test your salt sensitivity

If you'd like to know if you're salt-sensitive, you can try this three-step test.

1. Record your blood pressure and salt intake under normal circumstances.
2. Restrict salt to 2,000 mg a day and record your blood pressure.
3. Increase salt by 1,000 mg a day to determine when more salt causes your blood pressure to rise.

People with high blood pressure, African Americans, and the elderly are more likely to be salt sensitive. If you discover that you are salt sensitive, lowering your salt intake to around 500 mg a day, about one-quarter of a teaspoon, seems to be most effective.

&. &.

When a low-salt diet is dangerous

Although studies show cutting down on salt helps most people lower their blood pressure, a few have found the opposite. In some people, a low-salt diet actually increases blood pressure.

One study of 27 men found that some of the men with normal blood pressure were "salt-resistant," which means their blood pressure didn't automatically fall when they reduced their salt intake. In fact, blood pressure actually increased by as much as five points in some men who reduced their salt intakes.

Many of the men in the study had high levels of insulin, suggesting that the body may adapt to a low-salt diet by producing more insulin. Studies have shown that insulin sometimes contributes to hardening of the arteries by encouraging the body to produce excess cholesterol. Insulin also encourages your kidneys to retain salt.

If you have high blood pressure, and a low-salt diet doesn't seem to be helping you, talk with your doctor. You may be one of the few people who are salt-resistant.

👪 👪 👪

Watch out for sodium in your water

If you're on a severely sodium-restricted diet, your water may sabotage your efforts. If your home has a water softener, your water could contain extra sodium. Water softeners work by removing calcium, magnesium, and iron and adding sodium. Although it is unlikely your water could contain enough sodium to be a health problem, if you're trying to cut down on salt, you may want to have your water tested. The American Heart Association recommends water with a sodium concentration less than 20 mg per liter.

👪 👪

How to uncover the salt hiding in your food

Most of the sodium in your diet doesn't come from your saltshaker. It's already in your food.

Salt is a common seasoning and preservative in prepackaged foods. Before you toss that convenience food into your shopping cart, read the label carefully. Sodium can add up quickly. For example, your bowl of cornflakes in the morning may contain over 200 mg of sodium. The bowl of soup you had for lunch had almost 2,000 mg. What about the ham and cheese sandwich you ate with your soup? The bread could have added 300 mg, the ham 400 mg, and the cheese another 400 mg. You've already taken in more than the 2,400 recommended milligrams, and you haven't even had dinner yet.

Foods you don't think of as salty can nevertheless be high in sodium. You know potato chips are salty, but check the label on your favorite canned soup or dessert. You might be surprised.

Food	Serving size	Sodium (mg)
Bacon	3 slices	303
Bread	1 slice wheat	148
Bread	1 slice white	135
Cheesecake	1 slice	376
Cola	12 oz can	50
Cornflakes	1 cup	239
Cottage cheese	1 cup lowfat	918
Diet cola	12 oz can	40
Ham	1 slice	405
Hot dog	1 beef	462
Ice cream	1 cup chocolate	100
Pickle	1 medium dill	833
Potato chips	8 oz bag	1,348
Soup (canned)	1 cup vegetable beef	1,915
Soup (canned)	1 cup chicken noodle	1,862

Beware of over-the-counter salt

Many popular over-the-counter medications, particularly antacids, contain sodium. Make sure you read labels carefully. These medications are sodium free.

Bayer Aspirin	Vanquish	Bufferin
Sudafed	CoTylenol	Tylenol
Comtrex	Sine-Aid	Coricidin
Robitussin-DM	Ecotrin	Sine-Off
Pepto-Bismol	Contac	Excedrin
Phillips' Milk of Magnesia	Nytol	Triaminic Syrup

Salt-free ways to spice up your life

You don't have to give up on flavor and eat bland, uninteresting foods just because your doctor told you to cut down on salt. On the contrary, this can be an opportunity to experiment with new spices and add more zest to your usual salt-and-pepper routine.

Garlic. This aromatic herb can flavor more than just spaghetti sauce. Add it to soups, salads, casseroles, and vegetables. In addition to being a good substitute for salt, garlic has health benefits of its own. Try fresh garlic or powdered, but don't use garlic salt. You'd be defeating your salt-cutting purposes. For more information, read the *Garlic* chapter.

Lemon juice. Instead of shaking on salt the next time you're cooking fish, meat, or poultry, try squeezing on some fresh lemon juice. Besides the citrus zing, you'll be adding vitamin C to your food as well.

Parsley. The flat-leafed or "Italian" type of parsley has a strong taste that's well-suited to cooking. Like its cousin the carrot, it's packed with vitamins and minerals — beta carotene, folate, and iron. Plus, it's brimming with flavonoids, powerful plant chemicals that may guard your arteries against cholesterol build-up and lower your blood pressure. Check with your doctor if you take blood-thinning medication like warfarin. The vitamin K in parsley may counteract the medicine's effects.

Sage. The name of this herb comes from the Latin word for "safe," because it was believed to have healing powers. It was used as both a flavoring and a medicine. Pork, poultry, and stuffings are often flavored with sage, and it's a common ingredient in sausage.

Onion. This bulb comes from the same plant family as garlic, and it has many of the same health benefits. It can also add lots of flavor to your salt-free cooking. Read the *Garlic* chapter for more information about onions.

Dill. This herb was considered a good luck charm by 1st-century Romans. Using it instead of salt might bring you good luck with your blood pressure. It tastes great in salads, vegetables, and sauces. Fresh dill loses its flavor during heating, so add it when your dish is almost finished cooking. Dill seed, on the other hand, has a stronger flavor that is actually enhanced by cooking.

Basil. This fragrant herb was called the "royal herb" by the ancient Greeks. The tasty green leaves are the basis of Italian pesto. Add it to salads, soups, stews, meats, and pasta dishes.

Thyme. A basic herb in French cooking, thyme adds flavor to soups, vegetables, meat, fish, poultry, and cream sauces.

Turmeric. This bright orange-yellow spice was used as perfume in Biblical times. Today, it's used to add color, flavor, and aroma to foods. It is usually a principal ingredient in curry, and it gives prepared mustard its bright yellow color. According to some studies, curcumin, an ingredient in turmeric, may help prevent the growth of colon tumors.

How to read a food label for sodium content

Sodium-free	Less than 5 mg per serving
Very low sodium	35 mg or less per serving
Low sodium	140 mg or less per serving
Reduced sodium	Reduced in sodium by at least 25 percent per serving compared with the regular version

Sodium by any other name is still sodium

A rose is a rose is a rose, and sodium by any other name can still raise your blood pressure. When you're reading labels in search of salt, watch out for these sodium-containing compounds.

Salt (sodium chloride). Used as a seasoning; also used in canning and preserving.

Monosodium glutamate (MSG). A flavor enhancer used in home and restaurant cooking and in many packaged, canned, and frozen foods.

Baking soda (sodium bicarbonate). Used to leaven breads and cakes; sometimes added to frozen vegetables so they will retain their bright color; used to relieve indigestion.

Baking powder. Used to leaven quick breads and cakes.

Disodium phosphate. Found in some quick-cooking cereals and processed cheeses.

Sodium alginate. Used in many chocolate milks and ice creams to make the texture smooth.

Sodium benzoate. Used as a preservative in many condiments, such as relishes, sauces, and salad dressings.

Sodium hydroxide. Used in food processing to soften and loosen the skins of ripe olives and certain fruits and vegetables.

Sodium nitrite. Used in cured meats and sausages.

Sodium propionate. Used in some pasteurized cheeses and in some breads and cakes to inhibit the growth of molds.

Sodium sulfite. Used to bleach certain fruits, such as maraschino cherries and glazed or crystallized fruits that are to be artificially colored; also used as a preservative in some dried fruits, such as prunes.

Tomato-Basil Salad

2 fresh tomatoes, sliced
1/4 red onion, sliced and separated into rings
2 tablespoons fresh basil leaves, washed and chopped
1/4 cup vinaigrette dressing (see *Canola oil and olive oil* chapter)

Combine all ingredients and chill for one hour before serving.

Makes 2 to 3 servings

Per serving: 146 Calories; 14g Fat (2g from saturated fat) (86% calories from fat); 1g Protein; 5g Carbohydrate; 0mg Cholesterol; 90mg Sodium

Low-Sodium Marinade

1/4 cup red wine vinegar
1/4 cup water
2 tablespoons Worcestershire sauce
1 tablespoon honey
2 cloves garlic, minced
1 teaspoon basil
1 teaspoon oregano
1 teaspoon thyme

Mix liquids and garlic.

Mix spices. Crush leaves slightly. Stir into liquid mixture.

Pour over meat, poultry, or fish in plastic bag.

Marinate up to 24 hours in refrigerator. Turn bag at least once to evenly distribute marinade.

Makes 4 servings

Per serving: 29 Calories; less than 1g Fat (2% calories from fat); 0g Protein; 8g Carbohydrate; 0mg Cholesterol; 85mg Sodium

Quick Chicken and Vegetable Soup

Try a cup of this easy homemade soup. Regular canned soups can have more than four times the sodium found in this recipe.

16 ounces low-sodium tomatoes, broken up
13 3/4 ounces no-salt-added chicken broth
1 tablespoon chopped onion
1/2 cup cooked and cubed chicken breasts without skin
10 ounces frozen vegetable medley
1/4 teaspoon thyme
1/8 teaspoon pepper
1/8 teaspoon salt

Combine tomatoes and broth. Heat to boiling.

Add onion; simmer for 5 minutes.

Add remaining ingredients. Cover and cook over low heat until vegetables are tender, about 10 minutes.

Makes 4 servings

Per serving: 102 Calories; 1g Fat (less than 1g from saturated fat) (7% calories from fat); 13g Protein; 15g Carbohydrate; 14mg Cholesterol; 341mg Sodium

Seasoned Crumb Coating

If you enjoy the flavor and texture of "oven-fried" poultry, meat, or fish, try this low-sodium coating mix and give your taste buds a treat.

1 cup corn flake crumbs
1 teaspoon chili powder
1 teaspoon paprika
1/2 teaspoon onion powder
1/4 teaspoon garlic powder
1/4 teaspoon pepper
Mix ingredients thoroughly
Preheat oven to 400 degrees F.

Place some of the crumb coating in a plastic bag.

Dip poultry, meat, or fish in water then place in bag. Shake well.

Place on a rack in a baking pan. Bake until done; bone-in chicken will take about 50 minutes.

Discard any crumbs left in bag, but store unused portion in tightly covered container.

Makes 6 servings

Per serving: 20 Calories; less than 1g Fat (6% calories from fat); 0g Protein; 4g Carbohydrate; 0mg Cholesterol; 44mg Sodium

Oriental Vegetable Stir-fry

For a quick and easy low-sodium idea, try this vegetable stir-fry. Use it as a side dish or as a main dish served over rice.

1 cup thinly sliced celery
1 cup snow peas, trimmed
1 teaspoon olive oil
2 cups sliced Chinese cabbage
1 cup sliced mushrooms
1/2 cup red pepper, cut in thin strips
1 1/2 teaspoons cornstarch
1/2 teaspoon fresh ginger root, minced
1/8 teaspoon garlic powder
1/2 cup no-salt-added chicken broth
1 teaspoon low-sodium soy sauce

Stir-fry celery and snow peas in hot oil for 2 minutes.

Add Chinese cabbage, mushrooms, and red pepper. Stir-fry until almost tender, about 5 minutes.

Mix cornstarch, ginger root, and garlic powder. Stir into chicken broth; add soy sauce and stir into vegetables. Cook, stirring constantly until just thickened — about 1 minute.

Serve immediately.

Makes 4 servings

Per serving: 49 Calories; 1g Fat (22% calories from fat); 4g Protein; 7g Carbohydrate; 0mg Cholesterol; 239mg Sodium

Tortilla Snacks

1/2 cup canned tomatoes, diced and drained
1/4 cup chopped green pepper
2 tablespoons chopped onion
1 1/2 tablespoons chopped green chilies
1/2 teaspoon oregano
1/2 cup shredded, part-skim milk mozzarella cheese
16 whole, baked, unsalted Tostitos

Mix vegetables and oregano.

Add 1 tablespoon of vegetable mixture to each chip. Sprinkle with 1/2 tablespoon of cheese.

Place chips on baking sheet and broil for 5 minutes or until cheese melts.

Microwave instructions:

Place chips in a microwave-safe glass baking dish. Microwave on high power for 30 to 40 seconds or until cheese melts.

Makes 4 servings

Per serving: 83 Calories; 3g Fat (2g from saturated fat) (30% calories from fat); 5g Protein; 10g Carbohydrate; 8mg Cholesterol; 142mg Sodium

Selenium

Bypass heart disease with powerful antioxidant

Although your body needs only small amounts of selenium, it's vital for heart health. This powerful antioxidant helps keep your heart pumping oxygen-rich blood to every part of your body.

It does this by helping to form prostaglandins, hormone-like fatty acids that can help lower blood pressure and prevent blood clots. It also neutralizes free radicals, unstable molecules that damage cells through a process called oxidation. If left unchecked, free radicals would oxidize all your LDL cholesterol, making it even more damaging to your arteries. The more your arteries are damaged, the more plaque builds up on them and the narrower they become. Your heart must work harder and your chance of developing life-threatening blood clots is greater. But antioxidants, like selenium, keep this from happening. Many studies have shown that people who eat foods rich in antioxidants have a lower risk of heart disease.

Selenium is a mineral found naturally in most soils. In the course of various soil studies around the world, researchers realized that parts of the Carolinas and Georgia are extremely low in selenium. This area is sometimes referred to as the "stroke belt" because strokes and heart attacks are so common. They suspect a link between the low selenium levels and the large number of people with those serious illnesses.

A study in Denmark found that men with the lowest blood levels of selenium were 1.7 times more likely to suffer from heart disease. And in nearby Finland, a country plagued by heart disease, researchers found that people who had high blood selenium levels were 60 percent less likely to develop heart problems than those with low levels.

How to make sure you're getting enough

The best way to get more selenium is to eat a variety of foods and make smart choices, like choosing whole grains over refined foods. And don't overcook your vegetables. Boiling veggies reduces their selenium content by almost half. A high-sugar diet can also contribute to a selenium deficiency.

Most meats have adequate levels since the Department of Agriculture allows animal feed to be fortified with small amounts of selenium.

However, keep in mind that the selenium levels of vegetables, grains, and nuts can vary according to where they were grown. Generally, the Southeast and Northeast have the lowest levels of selenium. The Southwest has average selenium levels, and the Northwest, except for certain areas of the Pacific coast, the highest levels.

The recommended dietary allowance (RDA) for selenium is 70 micrograms (mcg) a day for adult men and 55 mcg for adult women.

Most experts don't recommend taking selenium supplements because too much may actually impair your immune system. Too much selenium can also be toxic.

One early sign of overdose is a metallic taste in your mouth. Other indicators include dizziness; diarrhea; nausea; persistent garlic breath; and loss of hair, nails, or teeth.

Best sources of selenium

whole grains	brown rice	fish	liver
beans and peas	soy products	Brazil nuts	brewer's yeast
broccoli	cabbage	celery	chicken
cucumbers	eggs	garlic	kidney
milk	mushrooms	radishes	seafood

Soy

Miracle bean slashes risk of heart disease

Soybeans contain plant hormones, or phytoestrogens, that are powerful weapons in the fight against heart disease and stroke. They lower cholesterol levels and help keep plaque from building up on the walls of your arteries. This enables your blood to flow freely.

In a major review of 38 clinical trials involving 730 volunteers, University of Kentucky researchers found that soybean eaters reduced their total cholesterol levels about 9 percent.

The study participants ate approximately 47 grams of soy protein per day — some ate more, some less — but all of them lowered their cholesterol levels. Volunteers with the highest cholesterol levels had the most dramatic results. They reduced their total cholesterol levels by nearly 20 percent. It seemed the more soy they ate, the more their cholesterol dropped.

Even better, the soy protein reduced only low-density lipoprotein cholesterol (LDL), the so-called "bad" cholesterol. Levels of high-density lipoprotein cholesterol (HDL), the "good" cholesterol, remained the same and sometimes increased.

For you to get 47 grams of soy protein, the amount used in the study, you would have to eat 14.5 ounces of tofu, drink almost 5 cups of soy milk, or bake with 3.6 ounces of soy flour every day.

If that sounds overwhelming, start slowly by substituting one soy meal a week for a meal based on animal protein. Over time, try to replace 50 percent of the animal protein you now eat with vegetable protein. Look in bookstores and libraries for cookbooks specializing in vegetarian, bean, and tofu cooking.

To make the most of soy's benefits, cut out the saturated fat in your diet, maintain a healthy weight, and exercise regularly.

Understand the dangers of soy

A few years ago, Dr. Lon White and his fellow researchers at the Pacific Health Research Institute in Hawaii examined the eating patterns of more than 8,000 Japanese-American men over a period of 30 years.

They found that those who ate two or more servings of tofu a week were far more likely to have memory problems as they got older than those who ate little or no tofu. And the more tofu they ate, the greater their memory and learning difficulties.

White suggests you eat soy only in moderate amounts.

9 ways to dish up some good-for-you soy

A few years ago, if you had a yen for soybean products, you could only find them in health food stores or Asian markets. Now, most supermarkets stock tofu and tempeh among the fresh produce, while other soy items are found in the health food section.

Although lower in fat, especially in saturated fat, than most animal proteins, soybeans still contain 19 percent polyunsaturated fat. To keep those fat grams under control, look for the low-fat soy products that are available, like low-fat soy milk and tofu.

Your goal is to replace high-fat, low-fiber meats with soy-based foods. Don't just add soy products to a typical high-protein American diet. If you add protein-rich soybeans to a meat-heavy diet, you're likely to have kidney trouble. Your kidneys will have to work overtime to excrete all the waste that is produced when your body metabolizes protein.

Experiment with the many varieties of soy products on the market. By eating soy instead of meat and dairy foods, you'll be giving your body extra firepower against high cholesterol, and you'll be reaping the benefits of a low-fat diet, as well.

Tofu. Besides soy sauce, tofu is probably the most well-know soybean product. You can use it as a substitute wherever meat, cheese, or yogurt is called for. Or simply add a few cubes to a recipe to give it an extra, healthful kick.

Sold in small blocks, this creamy, high-protein soybean curd is extremely rich in calcium. Look for "calcium sulfate" on the label for even more calcium. This is particularly important if you plan to replace cheese, milk, or yogurt in a recipe.

Since tofu comes in several textures, ranging from soft to extra firm, be sure to buy the right kind for the type of cooking you want to do. For example, extra firm tofu works best for grilling, while softer varieties are better suited for blending into dressings. Use it in soups, salads, stir-fries, dips, spreads, and even in thick milkshakes and cheesecake. Slice it, dice it, grate it, or mash it. Eat it raw, steamed, broiled, fried, or baked. One of the remarkable properties of tofu is that it has almost no taste. Instead, the tofu absorbs the flavor of whatever it is cooked with or marinated in.

Tofu is not necessarily low fat. A 3-ounce serving can have up to 9 grams of fat and anywhere from 50 to 145 calories. But if you're label conscious, you'll be able to find low-fat varieties.

Tofu is quite perishable. Choose fresh-looking tofu sold in dated, sealed, refrigerated packages and heat for two minutes in boiling water before using it. Avoid buying tofu from markets where it is left in unrefrigerated trays of water. That's an open invitation to high levels of bacteria. At home, tofu will keep in your refrigerator for up to a week. Store the tofu submerged in water, and change the water once a day.

Tempeh. Tempeh is another popular soy product that is a useful meat substitute. It is made from cooked, fermented soy-beans and contains even more protein than tofu. It comes in a firmer, cake-like form and has a slightly stronger flavor than tofu.

Tempeh can be grilled, stir-fried, served as shish kebab, or simply served plain. You can slice it; make it into patties; or dice it and add to chili, sloppy joes, burgers, stews, or stir-fries. It can be refrigerated for up to 10 days or frozen for as long as two months. A 3 1/2 ounce serving has about 200 calories; 8 grams of fat; and is rich in calcium, iron, and vitamin B12.

Tempeh is a little less common than tofu. You might have to visit a health food store or Japanese market to find it.

Soy milk. Made from cooked, ground soybeans, soy milk is available in low-fat versions and in powdered and flavored forms. Substitute it for dairy milk in cooking and baking, or pour it on cereal or into a tall glass and enjoy. Try mixing it 50-50 with low-fat or skim regular milk at first. Soy milk could be your easiest way to enjoy soy's benefits.

Miso. A salty seasoning paste rich in B-complex vitamins and iron, miso is made from fermented soybeans and grains, such as rice or barley. It has a distinct flavor that makes a tasty soup base or seasoning, but its sodium content is very high, so use it in moderation. Miso is an ingredient in some instant soups and ramen noodle products. You can make your own tasty, healthful treat by melting miso to taste in hot water and adding some diced green onion. It comes in an assortment of colors, tastes, and saltiness. Refrigerated, it keeps indefinitely. Better health food stores might carry it, but you'll probably have to visit an Oriental market to get your hands on some miso.

Soy cheese. Similar to tofu, but with a firmer texture, soy cheese comes in flavors like cheddar, mozzarella, and spiced jack. Keep it refrigerated.

Soy flour. Made from finely ground roasted soybeans, soy flour is a great way to boost the protein content of your home-cooked breads, muffins, and cakes. To enhance its natural nutty flavor, "toast" it in a dry skillet over medium heat for a few minutes before adding it to your recipe. Substitute soy flour for up to one-quarter of the flour called for in recipes for baked goods, but don't use only soy flour in recipes that include yeast. It doesn't have any gluten, which helps make the dough rise properly.

Ready for a new egg substitute? One tablespoon of soy flour plus one tablespoon of water equals one whole egg, but with no cholesterol or saturated fat.

Powdered soy protein. Powdered soy protein is available at almost all health food stores and can be mixed into juices, milk, yogurt, and just about anything else. While powdered protein does give you many of the benefits of soy, it does not carry the full nutritional value of soybeans. In addition, it hasn't been proven to lower cholesterol or reduce blood clotting, both heart disease risk factors.

Texturized vegetable protein (TVP). Made from compressed soy flour, TVP has a texture similar to ground beef and can be substituted for all or a portion of ground beef in your regular recipes. It is high in protein, calcium, iron, and zinc but low in calories and fat.

Meatless meat. New soy products include mock bacon, sausage, hot dogs, turkey, chicken, and beef. Some products even have a smoked taste. Watch out for high levels of sodium and fat by checking the labels.

More than 2,000 new soy foods were introduced in the last decade. The technology exists at this time to add soy to hot dogs, brownies, blueberry muffins, and ice cream without an unpleasant "beany" taste. And soy is already used in baby formulas and in some commercial baked goods, but not in high enough amounts to be beneficial.

Many researchers are hoping that the latest studies in heart disease, cancer, and osteoporosis will spur the public to demand more soy products from food companies.

🐜 🐜 🐜

Tempting ways with tofu

- Toss cubes of firm tofu into salads and stir-fries, or use it in place of meat in soups, stews, or chili. Add it during the last 15 minutes of cooking.

- Use silky tofu in place of ricotta cheese in homemade lasagna.

- Marinate extra-firm tofu in your favorite barbecue or teriyaki sauce, and grill it with onions and other vegetables.

- Mix 8 ounces of soy protein powder with one-half cup water and one-third cup frozen piña colada or other drink mix.

- Make a soy burger. Mix one-half cup texturized vegetable protein granules with two tablespoons cold water and 1 pound of lean ground beef. Knead, form into patties, and cook.

🐜 🐜

Tofu and Veggie Stir-fry

2 cups tofu, cubed
2 tablespoons olive oil
3/4 cup chopped onion
1 cup green pepper, cut in strips
1 cup sliced mushrooms
1/4 cup low-sodium soy sauce
1 1/4 cups bean sprouts
1/2 cup bamboo shoots
2 1/2 tablespoons cornstarch

Heat olive oil in a large skillet. Add green pepper and onions and cook until onion is translucent.

Add mushrooms and cook until tender, about 2 minutes. Scoop out vegetables from the pan and set aside.

Add tofu to the skillet and brown. Add sautéed vegetables to tofu mixture, including bean sprouts and bamboo shoots.

In a small bowl, blend soy sauce and cornstarch and pour into skillet. Cook for several minutes and serve over rice.

Makes 4 servings

Per serving: 189 Calories; 12g Fat (2g from saturated fat) (52% calories from fat); 11g Protein; 13g Carbohydrate; 0mg Cholesterol; 605mg Sodium

Tea

Powerful healing from a simple leaf

Steaming hot, soothingly warm, or icy cold — tea is one of the most popular beverages in the world, second only to water.

According to legend, in 2737 B.C., a servant of the Chinese emperor was boiling drinking water under a tree when a leaf fell in the water. The emperor decided to drink the brew anyway. The tree, of course, was a wild tea tree, and a new beverage was born.

Tea soon earned a reputation for possessing special healing powers. It was introduced in Japan as a medicine from China. The ancient Orientals may have been right on the mark with their medicinal tea.

Several studies have confirmed tea's ability to protect against various diseases, including heart disease and stroke. One study found that men who drank more than 4.7 cups of tea a day had a 69 percent reduced risk of stroke, compared with those who drank less than 2.6 cups a day. Another study found that Japanese men who drank 10 cups or more of green tea a day had lower levels of total cholesterol and LDL cholesterol.

Scientists have found that tea is chock full of flavonoids, substances in plants that protect against disease. One study found that LDL cholesterol exposed to tea flavonoids was less likely to become oxidized, which makes it more damaging to your arteries. Tea also reduces your blood's clotting abilities, which may help prevent heart attacks and strokes.

However it works, tea seems to do your heart good, so drink up.

A consumer's guide to tea

Sipping a soothing beverage to help your heart may be just your cup of tea, but with so many blends and brands available, you may be confused about which brew to buy.

All real tea comes from the same type of plant, *Camellia sinensis*, which can be either a shrub or a tree, depending on the variety. The three types of teas are green, black, and oolong.

To get green tea, the leaves are just picked and steamed — almost no processing at all. This means it retains more flavonoids than black tea, which is processed a lot longer and allowed to ferment. Oolong tea is somewhere in between the two. Although both green tea and black tea have proven health benefits, green tea is clearly the healthier winner.

There are many varieties and blends of these three types of tea. Some are named for the region in which they are grown, like Darjeeling, named after a mountain region in India. Earl Grey, a blend of black tea and bergamot oil, is named after a prime minister of England. Experiment with different blends until you find one you like.

You've probably seen lots of herbal teas in your grocery store, but most herbal teas don't contain real tea. Check the label. If it doesn't list "tea" in the ingredients, it's not the type of tea that scientists claim protects against heart disease. That doesn't mean herbal teas aren't healthy. Many herbs have health claims of their own.

Once you've picked out your tea, follow these four golden rules to brew a really good cup.

- Prerinse the teapot or teacup you'll be using for your tea with hot water.

- Fill your tea kettle with fresh, cold water. Reheated water gives tea a flat taste. Bring water to a rolling boil. If you're brewing green tea, remove the kettle from the heat and let it sit with the lid open for a few minutes. Green tea needs to be steeped at cooler temperatures than black or oolong teas. For black tea, use water immediately.

- Use one tea bag or 1 teaspoonful of tea for every cup of water. Pour water over the tea. With loose tea, you normally start with 1 teaspoonful of tea. To see what taste suits you best, experiment with different amounts, more or less.

- Watch the clock. Tea should be brewed for three to five minutes. The color of tea is not a good indicator of its strength. If you find that the tea is too strong for you after it's finished brewing, add a little warm water.

🍵 🍵 🍵

Advertisement for tea — 1657

Tea's reputation for healing goes way back. In 1657, a London advertisement claimed that tea "helpeth the Headache, giddiness, and heavyness thereof; it removeth the obstructions of the Spleen; it is good against Crudities, strengthening the weakness of the Ventricle or Stomack, causing good Appetite and Digestion, and particularly for Men of a corpulent Body, and such as are great eaters of Flesh, it vanquishes heavy dreams, easeth the Brain, and strengtheneth the Memory. It overcometh superfluous Sleep and prevents Sleepiness in general, a draught of the Infusion being taken so that without trouble whole nights may be spent at study without hurt to the Body, in that it moderately heateth and bindeth the mouth of the Stomack (it being prepared with Milk and Water), strengtheneth the inward parts, and prevents Consumptions, and powerfully assuages the pains of the Bowels, or griping of the Guts and Loosening."

Tomatoes

Delicious way to cut heart attack risk in half

Don't feel too guilty the next time you indulge in a thick slice of pizza or a steaming bowl of spaghetti — especially if you order it with extra sauce. Researchers say you'll be doing your heart a favor.

Tomatoes contain lycopene, a compound that not only gives certain foods their red coloring but also works like an antioxidant. Antioxidants protect your arteries from damage caused by unstable molecules called free radicals. Researchers found that men eating large amounts of lycopene had about half the risk of heart attack as other men. Even beta-carotene, another powerful antioxidant, doesn't afford this much protection.

Although experts believe it is better to get lycopene naturally by eating foods like tomatoes, they are conducting tests with lycopene supplements to find out how else lycopene can aid your body. They found that 60 milligrams (mg) of lycopene a day for three months dropped bad LDL cholesterol levels a whopping 14 percent. You would need to eat a little over 2 pounds of fresh tomatoes or a little less than 4 ounces of tomato paste to get this amount of lycopene.

Tired of tomatoes? Don't worry — there are other foods rich in lycopene that will make your daily menu a bit more interesting. Try watermelon, red grapefruit, guava, papaya, and apricots.

Since tomatoes contain the most lycopene, eat them often. For maximum heart protection, eat your tomatoes cooked and drizzle just a bit of olive oil on them. Cooking releases the lycopene, and the oil makes it more easily absorbed. Tomato paste, being both cooked and more concentrated, is an excellent source of lycopene, but any tomato product will do — even ketchup.

Tomatoes are also a rich source of vitamins A, C, E, and folic acid, as well as the mineral potassium — all heart-saving nutrients.

Food (100 grams)	Lycopene (mg)
Ketchup	9.9
Tomato juice, canned	8.6
Tomato paste, canned	6.5
Tomato sauce, canned	6.3
Guava, fresh	5.4
Watermelon, fresh	4.1
Papaya, fresh	3.7
Grapefruit, pink	3.4
Guava juice	3.3
Tomatoes, fresh, raw	2.9
Apricots, dried	0.86
Apricots, canned	0.07
Apricots, fresh	0.005

Heart Lover's Italian Sauce

1 pound ground turkey
2 tablespoons olive oil
1 onion, chopped
2 cloves garlic, minced
28 ounces canned chopped tomatoes
28 ounces canned tomato puree
2 tablespoons oregano, chopped
1 tablespoon fresh basil, chopped
1 cup dry red wine
black pepper to taste

In large pan sauté onion and garlic in olive oil. Cook until onion is transparent.

Add ground turkey and brown until it is no longer pink.

Drain any fat from the pan and add remaining ingredients. Simmer on low heat for about 1 hour. Use in lasagna or over spaghetti.

Makes 8 servings

Per serving: 205 Calories; 9g Fat (2g from saturated fat) (40% calories from fat); 13g Protein; 17g Carbohydrate; 45mg Cholesterol; 153mg Sodium

Use this low-fat version for spaghetti or lasagna.

Halibut Italiano

Great dish and easy to prepare. Other types of white fish may be substituted.

1 1/2 pounds halibut fillets cut into 4 servings
2 cups prepared spaghetti sauce
1/2 cup sliced mushrooms
1/4 cup sliced olives
1/2 cup mozzarella or cheddar cheese
olive oil

Place fish in oiled baking pan. Top with mushrooms and olives.

Pour spaghetti sauce over the top and bake for 10 minutes at 400 degrees F.

Remove from oven and sprinkle with cheese. Bake 10 more minutes or until fish flakes easily with a fork.

Serve with chopped parsley over the top and a lemon wedge on the side.

Makes 4 servings

Per serving: 375 Calories; 13g Fat (3g from saturated fat) (32% calories from fat); 42g Protein; 21g Carbohydrate; 62mg Cholesterol; 865mg Sodium

Reprinted with permission from the Alaska Seafood Marketing Institute www.state.ak.us/local/akpages/COMMERCE/asmihp.htm

Deep-Days-of-Summer Gazpacho

This classic summer soup is a delicious powerhouse of vegetables. It provides each person with about two and a half vegetable servings!

4 cups low-sodium tomato juice
1 small onion, minced
2 cups fresh tomatoes, diced
1 cup minced green pepper
1 teaspoon honey
1 clove garlic, crushed
1 diced cucumber
2 scallions, chopped
juice of 1/2 lemon and 1 lime
2 1/2 tablespoons balsamic vinegar
dash of cumin
1/2 cup fresh parsley, chopped
dash of hot pepper sauce
1 tablespoon olive oil
salt and pepper to taste

Combine all ingredients and chill for at least two hours. This soup can also be blended, if desired.

Makes 6 servings

Per serving: 100 Calories; 3g Fat (less than 1g from saturated fat) (22% calories from fat); 4g Protein; 19g Carbohydrate; 0mg Cholesterol; 138mg Sodium

This is an official 5 A Day Recipe. This recipe is provided by the National Institutes of Health.

Veggie Volley Bowl

When it comes to a low-fat, low-cost, all-in-one meal, this is a hands-down favorite. It's ready in half an hour, perfect for busy weeknights.

2 tablespoons olive oil
1 medium onion, chopped
1 zucchini, sliced
1 eggplant, chopped into small cubes
15 ounces chunky-style stewed tomatoes with herbs and garlic
15 ounces white cannelli beans, drained and rinsed
1 1/2 cups white rice or 1 10-ounce box plain couscous*

Heat oil in a large saucepan or wok. Add chopped onion and cook at medium-high heat until translucent, about 5 minutes.

Add zucchini and eggplant and cook about 5 minutes more. Add tomatoes, including liquid, and beans to vegetable mixture and simmer until heated through, about 10 minutes.

Meanwhile, prepare rice or couscous according to directions on box. Remove vegetables from heat and serve over couscous, along with salad and bread.

* Couscous is a starch made from semolina that's very fast and easy to prepare. It is available in most grocery stores, near the rice and pasta.

Makes 6 servings

Per serving: 487 Calories; 6g Fat (1g from saturated fat) (10% calories from fat); 22g Protein; 90g Carbohydrate; 0mg Cholesterol; 288mg Sodium

This is an official 5 A Day Recipe. This recipe is provided by the National Institutes of Health.

Vitamin A

Pick deep orange and dark green for heart health

The next time you go grocery shopping, fill up your cart with colorful fruits and vegetables. The deeper and richer the color, the more beta carotene the food is likely to have. Beta carotene is a carotenoid, a substance found in plants, that turns into vitamin A in your body.

Vitamin A and beta carotene protect your heart by fighting free radicals, those pesky molecules that can make bad LDL cholesterol even worse.

In one study, a large group of male doctors with heart disease took 50 milligrams (mg) of beta carotene every other day. Compared with men who didn't take beta carotene, they had almost half the number of heart attacks and strokes. Although, it took two years of taking supplements before the men saw any positive results.

A study of nearly 1,300 elderly Massachusetts residents had similar results, as did the Nurses' Health Study, with a smaller dosage. Women who ate more than 15 to 20 mg of beta carotene a day had a 40 percent lower risk of stroke and a 22 percent lower risk of heart attack, as compared with women who ate less than 6 mg a day.

Vitamin A performs many important functions in your body besides protecting your heart. It is essential for good eyesight, healthy skin, proper bone growth, and a strong immune system so you can fight infections. Vitamin A exists in several forms in your body, including retinol, retinal, and retinoic acid, collectively called retinoids.

The recommended dietary allowance (RDA) for vitamin A is expressed in retinol activity equivalents (RAE). This is the amount of retinol your body gets from foods containing vitamin A. However, you may sometimes see vitamin A amounts listed in international units (IU) on some food labels.

Recommended dietary allowance (RDA)

Males over 50	900 mcg RAE	3,000 IU
Females over 50	700 mcg RAE	2,300 IU

Vitamin A is a fat soluble vitamin. An extremely low-fat diet, or any disorder that interferes with fat absorption, can cause a deficiency. Diabetics may develop a deficiency because they don't convert carotene to retinol as well as most people.

Too much vitamin A can be dangerous. Because it is fat soluble, it can be stored in your body over long periods of time. This makes it easier for you to accumulate toxic amounts. Vitamin A overdose can cause vomiting, headaches, bone abnormalities, and joint pain. Extremely high doses (five times or more over the RDA) can cause irreversible or fatal liver damage. Because of this, most doctors don't recommend taking vitamin A supplements.

Unless you eat liver every day, it is virtually impossible to get too much vitamin A from your diet. And the only side effect of too much beta carotene in your diet is yellowish skin.

Food sources of vitamin A

Food	Amount	Vitamin A
Apricot	3 medium	276 RAE
Beef liver	3 ounces, fried	9,120 RAE
Broccoli	1 cup cooked	216 RAE
Butter	1 tablespoon	107 RAE
Cantaloupe	1/2 melon	859 RAE
Carrot	1 medium	2,025 RAE
Chicken liver	1 cup, cooked	6,878 RAE
Cottage cheese	1 cup	100 RAE
Milk	1 cup, whole	75 RAE
Spinach	1 cup, cooked	1,474 RAE
Tomato	1 medium	76 RAE

Salmon-Spinach Party Dip

1 can (7 1/2 ounces) Alaska salmon
10 ounces frozen chopped spinach, thawed and thoroughly
drained
1 cup plain nonfat yogurt
1/2 cup light mayonnaise
1/2 cup chopped parsley
1/2 cup chopped green onions
1/2 teaspoon dried basil
1/2 teaspoon dill weed
1/4 teaspoon grated lemon peel
assorted raw vegetables and crackers

Drain and flake salmon. Combine flaked salmon with remaining ingredients, except vegetables and crackers.

Chill several hours to blend flavors. Serve dip with vegetables and crackers.

Makes 16 servings, about 4 cups

Per serving (not including vegetables and crackers): 39 Calories; 1g Fat (less than 1g from saturated fat) (29% calories from fat); 4g Protein; 3g Carbohydrate; 11mg Cholesterol; 136mg Sodium

Reprinted with permission from the Alaska Seafood Marketing Institute www.state.ak.us/local/akpages/COMMERCE/asmihp.htm

Cantaloupe Crush

This refreshing drink provides each person served with 1 serving of fruit.

1/2 cantaloupe
1 cup fat-free milk
1 1/2 cups ice
1 to 2 teaspoons of sugar or the equivalent in artificial sweetener (optional)

Cut cantaloupe into small cubes.

Blend all ingredients until smooth. Sweeten to taste.

Makes 4 servings

Per serving: 41 Calories; less than 1g Fat; 2g Protein; 8g Carbohydrate; 1mg Cholesterol; 37mg Sodium

This is an official 5 A Day Recipe. This recipe provided by the National Institutes of Health.

Arizona Grown Recipe — Carrot Raisin Salad

4 medium carrots, shredded
1/4 cup raisins
2 teaspoons sugar
juice of 1 lemon

In a medium bowl, thoroughly mix carrots, raisins, sugar, and lemon.

Serve chilled.

Makes 4 servings

Per serving: 78 Calories; less than 1g Fat; 1g Protein; 21g Carbohydrate; 0mg Cholesterol; 24mg Sodium

This is an official 5 A Day Recipe. This recipe provided by the National Institutes of Health.

Vitamin C

Powerful antioxidant battles heart disease

You know how sliced apples and potatoes turn brown if you leave them on your kitchen counter too long? Exposure to oxygen in the air causes them to change color. This process, called oxidation, can also damage cells in your body.

As your body processes oxygen, it produces chemicals called free radicals. These free radicals are molecules that are unstable because they lack an electron. They travel through your body like a band of pickpockets, trying to steal electrons from healthy cells. When they succeed, they leave the cell permanently damaged. One damaged cell will not usually cause your body much distress. But over time, lots of these pickpocket molecules can cause so much damage your body becomes weak and more likely to fall prey to heart disease and cancer.

Luckily, your body also produces antioxidants, which neutralize free radicals. Antioxidants fight oxidation by combining with free radicals to form a harmless substance or by contributing an electron to the free radical, making it stable.

Research indicates that vitamin C may be a particularly effective antioxidant against heart disease. One large study found that men with the highest intake of vitamin C had almost a 50 percent lower death rate from heart disease. Researchers aren't sure if vitamin C was the cause of this lower rate, or if people who get lots of vitamin C just tend to have other heart-healthy habits, too.

However, vitamin C does seem to improve factors associated with good heart health. Studies find it raises HDL cholesterol, which is considered to be protective against heart disease, and it helps prevent LDL cholesterol from becoming oxidized and turning into artery-clogging plaques. High levels of vitamin C are also associated with lower blood pressure, and it helps keep your small blood vessels springy and healthy.

Vitamin C may even help you recover after a heart attack. One study found that people who ate a lot of vitamin C-rich foods while recovering from a heart attack had lower levels of an enzyme that is an indicator of heart damage.

The current recommended dietary allowance (RDA) for vitamin C is 90 milligrams (mg) daily for men over 50 and 75 mg for women over 50. This isn't difficult to get from your diet. If you choose to take supplements, be aware that some supplements contain as much as 1,000 mg or even more. Although too much vitamin C probably won't kill you, large doses may cause kidney stones, nausea, abdominal cramps, and diarrhea. A recent study found that the body has trouble absorbing more than 400 mg at a time, so if you take more than that, you may just lose the rest in your urine. Your best bet is to eat more fruits and vegetables. If you eat the recommended five servings of fruits and vegetables a day, you're probably getting about 200 mg of vitamin C daily.

Food sources of vitamin C

Sweet red peppers, 1 raw	226 mg
Orange juice, 1 cup	120 mg
Green peppers, 1 raw	106 mg

Kiwifruit, 1 medium	98 mg
Strawberries, 1 cup	86 mg
Cantaloupe, 1 cup	66 mg
Brussels sprouts, 1/2 cup	48 mg
Tomato juice, 1 cup	45 mg
Grapefruit, 1/2 medium	44 mg
Collard greens, 1 cup	35 mg
Broccoli, 1 spear	28 mg
Cabbage, raw, 1 cup	22 mg

Funny-looking fruit loaded with vitamin C

Ounce for ounce, what fruit contains the most vitamin C? If you said an orange, you'd be wrong. That honor belongs to a fuzzy little fruit you should eat more often — the kiwifruit.

When comparing kiwis and oranges, the kiwi comes out ahead more than 2 to 1. One orange contains about 45 mg of vitamin C, but one kiwifruit contains about 98 grams of vitamin C.

Kiwi is also loaded with potassium, another important nutrient in the battle against heart disease.

These interesting fruits are also known as Chinese Gooseberries. They originated in the Chang Kiang Valley of China, where they were a favorite of the ancient Khans. Later, New Zealand farmers scored a marketing coup when they grew this fruit successfully and then renamed it the "kiwi fruit" after their national bird.

Holiday Kiwifruit Salad

1 pear, cored and cubed
1 red apple, cored and thinly sliced
lemon or lime juice
1 can (8 ounces) jellied cranberry sauce, divided
2 California kiwifruit, pared and sliced
red leaf lettuce
1/3 cup light sour cream

Dip pear and apple in lemon juice to prevent darkening.

Reserve 3 tablespoons cranberry sauce; slice remainder into quarter slices.

Arrange kiwifruit, cranberry sauce slices, pear, and apple on lettuce.

For dressing, combine sour cream with 3 tablespoons reserved cranberry sauce and 1 teaspoon lemon juice.

Makes 4 or 5 servings

Per serving: 125 Calories; 1g Fat (0g from saturated fat) (5% calories from fat); 1g Protein; 31g Carbohydrate; 1mg Cholesterol; 19mg Sodium

Reprinted with permission from the California Kiwifruit Commission

Tropical Eye-Openers

1 large, ripe mango
1 large banana
1 cup 100 percent grapefruit juice
1/2 cup nonfat vanilla frozen yogurt
1/8 teaspoon grated nutmeg
1 1/2 cups ice
1 to 2 teaspoons sugar or the equivalent in artificial sweetener
(optional)

Peel the mango over a bowl to catch the juices. Then, use a
paring knife to slice the flesh away from the stone.

Add all ingredients to blender container. Blend until smooth.

Sweeten to taste.

Makes 4 servings

Per serving: 379 Calories; 1g Fat (less than 1g from saturated fat)
(2% calories from fat); 7g Protein; 92g Carbohydrate; 0mg
Cholesterol; 81mg Sodium

This is an official 5 A Day Recipe. This recipe is provided by the National
Institutes of Health.

Vitamin E

Powerful antioxidant zaps cholesterol

Picture your healthy blood vessels, with smooth, slick walls — wide enough for blood to slide through easily. Now picture those same blood vessels narrowed by arterial plaques sticking to the walls, blocking blood flow and slowing it down on its way to bring nourishment to your body. That's what happens when bad LDL cholesterol becomes oxidized by free radicals.

Free radicals are rogue molecules, formed from oxygen, that attack healthy cells. When LDL is attacked by free radicals, its cholesterol becomes oxidized and is scavenged by your immune system's white blood cells. The result is what's known as foam cells. These foam cells stick to your blood vessel walls, the first step in creating those artery-clogging plaques.

Fortunately, you have powerful ammunition to use against free radicals. This ammunition, known as antioxidants, fights oxidation by combining with free radicals to form a harmless substance. And, according to the latest research, vitamin E may be the most powerful antioxidant.

Vitamin E is particularly effective in protecting fats from becoming oxidized, perhaps because it is a fat-soluble vitamin.

Numerous studies have found that vitamin E can help protect your heart and blood vessels from free radical damage.

One study from the Harvard School of Public Health found that men who had taken at least 100 international units (IU) of vitamin E a day for at least two years had 37 percent fewer heart attacks than men who didn't take supplements. Another study found that women who took vitamin E supplements for more than two years had 41 percent fewer heart attacks.

Those studies were done on people who had no history of heart disease. The Cambridge Heart Antioxidant Study (CHAOS) was designed to find out if vitamin E could help people who already had heart disease.

Researchers gave the study participants 400 or 800 IU of vitamin E daily. After about 200 days of treatment, the participants' risk of having a nonfatal heart attack was reduced by 77 percent. Although the vitamin E didn't have an effect on death rates, the researchers pointed out that most deaths occurred early in the study, before the vitamin E would have had a chance to work.

Defend yourself from a life-threatening stroke

Vitamin E's ability to stop LDL cholesterol from clinging to your blood vessel walls may also help prevent another potential killer — stroke. The clots that form on artery walls sometimes break loose and travel to your brain where they can cause a stroke.

Vitamin E also fights stroke by making your blood more slippery and less likely to form clots. A study on the effects of another well-known anticoagulant, aspirin, found that people given 400 IU of vitamin E and 325 mg of aspirin to prevent blood clots were about half as likely to form clots as people taking aspirin alone.

🐝 🐝 🐝

An easy way to figure the RDA

The recommended dietary allowance (RDA) for vitamin E is 15 mg for men and women over 50.

To convert milligrams (mg) of vitamin E to international units (IU), multiply the mg by .67. For example, 15 mg x .67 = 10 IU.

🐝 🐝

How much do you really need?

You're convinced vitamin E is good for your heart. But should you take supplements, or do you get enough from your diet?

Most people get about 7 to 10 mg of vitamin E from foods daily, which is close to the RDA. However, most studies claiming heart benefits have used supplements at doses of 100 to 400 IU daily.

Certain conditions, such as smoking, increase your need for vitamin E. And while fish oil provides benefits of its own, be aware that taking fish oil supplements may increase your need for vitamin E.

Also keep in mind that most fat-soluble vitamins can cause serious side effects if taken in large quantities because they are stored in the body. Even though vitamin E seems to be relatively safe, taking large doses — more than 400 IU — over a prolonged period of time may cause blurred vision, diarrhea, dizziness, headaches, nausea, or unusual fatigue.

Be sure to check with your doctor before taking more than the RDA for vitamin E, especially if you're taking a blood thinning medicine like Coumadin.

Serve up some vitamin E

Natural sources of vitamin E include vegetable oils and related products like margarine, salad dressing, and shortening, although much of the vitamin E is lost if the oil has been heated to frying temperatures. Other sources include green leafy vegetables, wheat germ, whole-grain cereals, peanut butter, nuts, and eggs.

Check the following chart. It will show you how much vitamin E you're getting from the foods you eat.

Food	Amount	Vitamin E (mg)
Wheat germ oil	1 tablespoon	20
Almonds, dried	1 ounce	7
Sunflower seeds	1 ounce	6
Safflower oil	1 tablespoon	4.6
Avocado, California	1 medium	3.4
Mango	1 medium	2.3
Peanuts, dry roasted	1 ounce	2
Soybean oil	1 tablespoon	1.3
Sweet potato, baked	1 medium	.8
Spinach, raw	1 cup	.6
Mayonnaise	1 tablespoon	.3
Asparagus	4 spears	.2
Brown, rice, cooked	1 cup	.06

Mashed Sweet Potatoes

You may substitute 1/4 teaspoon cinnamon plus a dash of nutmeg and a dash of ginger for the pumpkin pie spice.

1 1/2 pounds sweet potatoes
1 1/2 tablespoons margarine, cut into pieces
1/2 teaspoon pumpkin pie spice

Scrub sweet potatoes thoroughly; cut off and discard small ends and inedible knobs. If large, cut into halves or thirds. Place in a deep cooking pot; add enough water to cover potatoes. Cover pot; bring to a boil. Cook over moderate heat until sweet potatoes are soft (about 25 minutes).

Drain at once. Hold each sweet potato with a fork, and peel quickly. Place potatoes in a bowl; mash. Beat in margarine and pumpkin pie spice.

Makes 6 servings

Per serving: 112 Calories; 3g Fat (.5g from saturated fat) (25% calories from fat); 1g Protein; 20g Carbohydrate; 0mg Cholesterol; 44mg Sodium

Reprinted with permission from The Art of Cooking for the Diabetic by Mary Abbott Hess, 1996

Sweet Potato Coins

*The liqueur is optional but adds a hint of almond flavor
and a bit of glaze.*

2 small (about 1 pound total) sweet potatoes
4 teaspoons margarine, melted
1 tablespoon amaretto, optional
1/4 teaspoon salt

Preheat oven to 400 degrees F. Peel sweet potatoes; cut cross-
wise into 1/4-inch slices. Spray a cookie sheet with nonstick
cooking spray. Spread sweet potato slices in a single layer on
pan. Brush tops with 2 teaspoons margarine and 1 1/2 teaspoons amaretto.

Bake sweet potatoes slices 10 minutes. Turn slices over; brush
tops with remaining 2 teaspoons margarine and 1 1/2 teaspoons amaretto. Bake another 10 minutes. Season with salt
and serve hot.

Makes 4 servings

Per serving: 130 Calories; 4g Fat (1g from saturated fat) (29%
calories from fat); 1g Protein; 21g Carbohydrate; 0mg
Cholesterol; 188mg Sodium

*Reprinted with permission from The Art of Cooking for the Diabetic
by Mary Abbott Hess, 1996*

Weight Loss

Put the bite on heart disease

You hold the answer to your heart's health — every time you lift a fork to your mouth. One of the best things you can do for your heart is to control your weight. Putting on a few extra pounds does more than just make it harder to button your jeans or zip your skirt. It also increases your odds of developing high blood pressure, high cholesterol, and diabetes, which contribute to heart disease. Recent research also indicates that being overweight can increase your risk of heart disease even if it doesn't cause any of those conditions.

Your heart is a muscle, and its job is to pump blood throughout your body. When you're overweight, you make its job much harder. Think about throwing a baseball. The farther you have to throw it, the more effort it takes. If you had to throw farther and farther, one baseball after another, you'd soon be worn out. When you're overweight, your heart has to work harder to pump blood over more territory.

Researchers estimate that a whopping 50 to 70 percent of heart disease cases are due to obesity. Believe it or not, that's actually good news. It means you have a lot of control over keeping your ticker healthy. According to a recent study, losing weight not only prevents heart disease, it may even correct some existing heart abnormalities.

Obese people tend to have abnormal left ventricles, the chamber that pumps oxygen-rich blood to all parts of the body. Researchers found that weight reduction not only reduced blood pressure, it led to favorable changes in the abnormal left ventricles.

Don't wait until you have heart problems to lose weight. The longer you carry that excess weight around, the more damage you can do to your heart. Maintain a healthy weight now and keep your heart steadily pumping for years to come.

The up side of yo-yo dieting

Have you experienced the ups and downs of weight cycling? If so, you may have heard that it's better to remain at a constant weight, even if that weight is roughly equivalent to that of a minivan. New studies, however, prove that weight cycling may not be so bad after all.

One reason weight cycling has gotten such a bad rap is that it supposedly has a negative effect on metabolism. A review of 43 studies on weight cycling revealed no evidence that the losing and regaining merry-go-round permanently lowers metabolism. The same review also found no connection between weight cycling and fat distribution or lean body mass. The main drawback to the ups and downs of weight loss could be the psychological effect — the harm to a dieter's self-esteem.

Another recent study on heart disease followed 153 overweight people for almost two and a half years. They were divided into groups who lost weight, gained weight, remained at a constant weight, or lost and regained. At the end of the study, those who lost weight had significantly reduced their risk factors for heart disease, while those who gained were at the greatest risk. The weight cyclers actually showed improvement in some risk factors when compared with those whose weight remained constant.

Of course, no one wants to keep losing the same 10 pounds over and over. But evidence indicates that it's just as easy to lose it the tenth time as it was the first, and you may be giving your heart a little boost. In the "weighting" game, even temporary losses seem to help, so if you can't stop the diet roller coaster at the bottom of a hill, just hold on tight and try again the next time around.

Trust your calculator, not your mirror

A mirror is a great tool for determining whether you have spinach stuck in your teeth, but it may not be your best tool for judging whether you need to lose weight. If you think the person in the mirror should be super-model thin, you may need a reality check. A more reliable method of determining how much you should weigh is the body mass index (BMI.)

Figuring out your BMI involves a little math, so you may want to have a calculator handy if you're mathematically challenged.

Step 1. Calculate your height in inches. For example, if you're 6'4" tall, this number would be 76.

Step 2. Square your height in inches. Using the above example, 76 squared (76x76) would be 5,776.

Step 3. Divide your weight in pounds by your squared height. Let's say you weigh 200 pounds. You would divide 200 by 5,776, which equals .035 (rounded off).

Step 4. Multiply the number you calculated in step 3 by 703. Using our example, your would multiply .035 by 703 to find the BMI, which in this case is 24.6 (rounded off).

A BMI of 19.1 to 25.8 is considered healthy for women, while a BMI of 25.8 to 27.3 is considered slightly overweight with some risk. If you're a woman, the higher your BMI goes above 27.3, the greater your health risk.

Because men generally have more muscle mass than women, their average BMIs are slightly higher. Men with a BMI of 20.7 to 26.4 are considered at low risk. A BMI of 26.4 to 27.8 is considered slightly overweight with some risk. If you're a man, the higher your BMI goes above 27.8, the greater your health risk.

If the math is too much for you, consult the following chart for approximate BMIs for common weights and heights. If you're too tall or too short for the chart, you'll have to rely on your trusty old calculator.

Weight

Height	100	110	120	130	140	150	160	170	180	190	200
5'0"	20	21	23	25	27	29	31	33	35	37	39
5'1"	19	21	23	25	26	28	30	32	34	36	38
5'2"	18	20	22	24	26	27	29	31	33	35	37
5'3"	18	19	21	23	25	27	28	30	32	34	35
5'4"	17	19	21	22	24	26	27	29	31	33	34
5'5"	17	18	20	22	23	25	27	28	30	32	33
5'6"	16	18	19	21	23	24	26	27	29	31	32
5'7"	16	17	19	20	22	23	25	27	28	30	31
5'8"	15	17	18	20	21	23	24	26	27	29	30
5'9"	15	16	18	19	21	22	24	25	27	28	30
5'10"	14	16	17	19	20	22	23	24	26	27	29
5'11"	14	15	17	18	20	21	22	24	25	26	28
6'0"	14	15	16	18	19	20	22	23	24	26	27
6'1"	13	15	16	17	18	20	21	22	24	25	26
6'2"	13	14	15	17	18	19	21	22	23	24	26
6'3"	12	14	15	16	17	19	20	21	22	24	25

Flatten your 'spare tire' for a healthy heart

Do you moan about having heavy hips and thunder thighs? Maybe you should count your blessings. Although excess weight is never good for you, researchers say where you carry your extra pounds can have a profound effect on your health.

People who are shaped like apples, with most of their extra fat in the abdominal area, are at higher risk for heart disease than pear-shaped people who carry their extra weight in their hips and behind them.

Researchers calculated waist-to-hip ratios (WHR) and found that a ratio greater than .85 in women and .95 in men was associated with higher blood pressure and other heart disease risk factors. One study suggested that WHRs might account for the difference in heart disease between men and women. Men are more likely to have heart disease than women. They are also more likely to carry their weight in their belly. When the study accounted for waist-to-hip ratios, the difference in heart disease rates between men and women virtually disappeared.

Another study found that a high WHR increased heart disease risk factors like blood pressure and cholesterol levels even in people who were not considered obese.

To figure out your waist-to-hip ratio, find a flexible measuring tape, like the ones seamstresses use. Measure your waist and your hips and divide your waist measurement by your hip measurement. For example, if your waist is 28 inches, and your hips are 40 inches, your waist-to-hip ratio would be 28 divided by 40, which is .70. If that were the case, you'd be in good shape for avoiding heart disease. If your numbers don't look that good, a healthy eating plan and regular exercise will melt away fat, including that spare tire around your middle.

Here's something else you could try ... relaxing. At least one researcher thinks it's possible to change your distribution of fat by learning to deal with stress.

Studies have found that people with high WHRs tend to have high levels of stress. A Swedish researcher thinks that an overabundance of a hormone called cortisol, which is released during times of stress, may cause fat to accumulate in your abdominal area.

Everyone has stress in their lives, but how you deal with it may make a difference. An attitude of helplessness is particularly associated with belly fat accumulation. Therapy or support groups may help some people learn to deal with their stress more effectively. If you're a do-it-yourselfer, bookstores and libraries have many self-help books that can give you pointers on calming down, taking control, and flattening that bulging belly.

Drop pounds to lower blood pressure

Does your blood pressure rise with your weight? It's not just the stress of seeing the numbers on your bathroom scale getting progressively higher. Excess weight is one of the main causes of high blood pressure, but here's the good news — dropping those extra pounds will lower your blood pressure. One study found that over 85 percent of people who were taking medicine to control their blood pressures were able to stop taking the medicine when they lost weight and controlled their salt and alcohol intake. Another study found that people who lost 10 pounds or more lowered their diastolic blood pressure (the bottom number) by an average of 12 points.

Weight loss tips that really work

If you want to lose weight, your options are practically endless. Walk into any bookstore. The shelves are filled with all kinds of self-help books. Open up your phone book. You'll see plenty of supervised weight loss programs like Weight Watchers and Overeaters Anonymous. Talk with your doctor and ask him for help. Whatever method you choose, these tips will help guarantee your success.

♦ **Get real.** Perhaps the first step to successful weight loss is to set realistic goals for yourself. If you're determined to lose 20 pounds in one week, you're setting yourself up for failure, and nothing will make you give up on a diet quicker than a big dose of failure. Instead, set goals you know you can reach. "I will walk 20 minutes every day." "I will eat less fat today." "When I am tempted to eat candy this week, I will eat a piece of fruit instead." These are the types of goals you have total control over.

♦ **Take your time.** Quick weight loss is usually temporary weight loss. If you want to take it off — and keep it off — you need to take your time. Shortcuts and fad diets usually don't work in the long run. You have to get rid of your unhealthy eating habits for good. Remember ... slow and steady wins the race.

♦ **Write it down.** Many weight loss champs have found that keeping a food diary can be helpful. It's important to know about how many calories you consumed during the day, and it's really easy to forget that bowl of ice cream you had after lunch. If you write down everything you eat and drink, you'll have a better idea of where you're having a problem.

♦ **Exercise.** Move it and you'll lose it. One of the best ways to get rid of those excess calories is to burn them off during exercise. It doesn't really matter what kind of exercise you do, as long as you find something you enjoy. If you're having fun, you're much more likely to stick with it. See the *Exercise* chapter for more information on how to keep it in motion.

6 sure-fire ways to lose weight

You've taken the first step. You've chosen an eating and exercise plan. But here's the bottom line — if you want to lose weight, you have to burn more calories than you take in. It takes 3,500 calories to make a pound of fat. That means in order for you to lose one pound, you have to burn 3,500 calories more than you take in. Here are some helpful hints for cutting those calories and getting rid of the fat.

◆ **Shop smart.** Look in your kitchen cupboards, and clean out all the junk food. Give it to your neighbors or throw it away, but get rid of anything that's not allowed on whatever food plan you chose. Then go shopping for healthy foods, like lots of fresh fruits and veggies. Make sure you eat before you go shopping so you won't be tempted by the wrong foods.

◆ **Pay attention.** You need to be in control of your food intake, and if you're not paying attention to what you're eating, you're not in control. Don't eat while you're standing up or doing other things. It's too easy to scarf down a pint of ice cream while watching a really intense horror movie. Suddenly, the movie is over, and you have an empty carton in your hands, and no idea how it got there.

◆ **Fill up with fiber.** That gnawing empty feeling in the pit of your stomach can sabotage your best weight loss efforts. You can avoid that empty feeling by making sure you get plenty of fiber. Fiber fills you up because it absorbs water and swells, taking up more space. Fiber also slows movement of your food through your upper digestive tract, so you don't get hungry again as quickly. Fill your diet with fiber-rich foods like whole-grains, fruits, vegetables, and legumes, and keep your stomach from growling at you.

- **Think small.** Thinking of yourself 25 pounds smaller is great motivation, but you should also think small in regard to meals. Small meals spaced out over the day keep you from getting too hungry and overindulging. Eating from a small plate is another old dieter's trick that may help.

- **Cook it right.** You can buy all the right foods, but if you cook them in fat, you'll add dozens of calories. Use low-fat cooking methods, like broiling, poaching, grilling, and baking instead of frying. Nonstick cookware can help you avoid adding too much fat to your foods.

- **Drink plenty of water.** Water is an essential nutrient necessary for digestion. You could live about 45 days without food, but without water, you would only last about 10 days. If you drink a tall glass of ice water before a meal, it dulls your appetite. That makes you less likely to overeat.

Maximize your weight loss efforts

If you're overweight, losing those extra pounds will improve your health in many ways, but be careful your weight loss efforts don't cause more harm than good. Here are some things not to do when you're trying to peel off those pounds.

- **Don't crash.** Crash diets are appropriately named because they can bring your metabolism crashing down. Being overweight may be unhealthy, but not eating enough to meet your daily nutritional needs can be worse. Crash diets aren't usually effective either, at least not in the long run. People who fast or go on very low calorie diets are much more likely to gain back the pounds they lost than people who follow a sensible diet with a slow and steady weight loss.

- **Don't wrap.** Elegant salons now offer body wraps to spot-reduce problem areas. It's an updated version of the plastic-wrap-around-the-thighs method of reducing. The problem with this is all you lose is sweat, not fat. The loss is a temporary one, and it can be harmful if your body temperature increases too much.

♦ **Don't take pills.** Diet pills should only be used under a doctor's supervision and usually only in cases of extreme obesity. Over-the-counter appetite suppressants may contain phenylpropanolamine hydrochloride (PPA), which may cause high blood pressure. If you have diabetes, heart disease, thyroid disease, or high blood pressure, you shouldn't use products containing PPA. Even if you don't have any of these conditions, think twice before buying these appetite suppressants. The Food and Drug Administration (FDA) is taking steps to remove PPA from all drugs and medications. In the meantime, they've asked drug companies to voluntarily stop marketing products that contain PPA or change their products to exclude this potentially dangerous ingredient. The FDA recommends you read labels before you buy.

Beware of those 'fat-free' calories

A package in the grocery store with "fat-free" on the front practically screams at you to buy it. There's just something about the word "free" that sounds so ... well, liberating. Modern technology has made it possible to remove the fat and keep all the taste and texture of your favorite goodies. So, with the astounding variety of fabulous fat-free foods available today, why are people still getting fat?

The answer is simple. Fat free doesn't mean calorie free. Some people actually gain weight when they start eating fat-free foods because they mistakenly believe they can eat as much fat-free foods as they want.

In one study, researchers gave women yogurt before lunch every day in a package that was either unlabeled or labeled "high-fat" or "low-fat." When the women ate from a package labeled "low-fat," they consumed more calories at the following lunch and dinner than they did when they ate the yogurt labeled "high-fat." Researchers think people feel so good about eating low-fat they reward themselves by eating more later. "I can have this slice of cheesecake — after all, I ate some low-fat yogurt earlier."

Your best protection against this syndrome is to be a scrupulous label reader. Don't just check for fat content. Keep reading until you find out how much sugar and calories are in there, too. Many fat-free foods are loaded with sugar to make up for the taste lost when the fat was removed.

For more healthy eating tips, see the *Low-fat eating* chapter.

🐜 🐜 🐜

Smashing diet myths

Fooled into eating too many calories by the abundance of fat-free foods? Don't feel too bad — the same syndrome occurred with artificial sweeteners in the 1980s. A 1982 American Cancer Society study found that dieters who used artificial sweeteners, like aspartame, which became available to the public in 1981, were more likely to gain weight than dieters who didn't use artificial sweeteners.

Researchers say people thought they were saving so many calories by using the artificial sweeteners they began consuming more calories than they did before. It is also possible that artificial sweeteners, which are actually sweeter than sugar, increased the dieters' desires for sweets.

More recent studies haven't found that artificial sweeteners increase hunger or contribute to weight gain. This may reflect the public's awareness of the "I drank a diet soda, so I can eat this candy bar" syndrome. People are now more knowledgeable about how to use artificial sweeteners to their benefit.

🐜 🐜

Index

(TVP) 331
Tofu 329
  recipe that contains 332-333
Tomatoes 339-340
  recipes that contain 110, 258-260, 316, 321, 341-344
Trans fatty acids 87, 90
Triglycerides 21
  low-fat eating and 262
Triticale 119
Type A personality 51
  estrogen and 184
Type D personality 52

V

Valerian 242-243
Ventricles 4
Vitamin A 345-347
  amounts in foods 347
  cautions 346
  recipes that contain 347-349
  recommended dietary allowance 346
Vitamin B12 79
  recommended dietary allowance 78
Vitamin B6 79
  recommended dietary allowance 78
Vitamin C 351-353
  amounts in foods 352-353
  recipes that contain 354-355
  recommended dietary allowance 352
Vitamin D
  in eggs 176
  recommended dietary allowance 176
Vitamin E 357-360
  amounts in foods 360
  recipes that contain 361-362

  recommended dietary allowance 359
VLDL (Very low density lipoprotein) 21. *See also* Cholesterol

W

Waist-to-hip ratios (WHR) 367
Walnuts 288
Water
  weight loss and 371
Water softeners
  sodium in 312
Weight loss 363-373
  chromium and 131
Wine 233. See also Alcohol
  in Mediterranean diet 165

Y

Yerba mate 141
Yoga 284
Yogurt
  recipes that contain 62, 100-102, 347

Z

Z-Trim
  recipes that contain 203
Zestril 42
Zocor 24